T0103235

MEDICINAL HERBS
OF WESTERN CANADA

Text and art by
BRENDA JONES

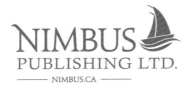
NIMBUS
PUBLISHING LTD.
—— NIMBUS.CA ——

Copyright © 2024, Brenda Jones

All rights reserved. No part of this book may be reproduced, stored in a retrieval system or transmitted in any form or by any means without the prior written permission from the publisher, or, in the case of photocopying or other reprographic copying, permission from Access Copyright, 1 Yonge Street, Suite 1900, Toronto, Ontario M5E 1E5.

Nimbus Publishing Limited
3660 Strawberry Hill Street, Halifax, NS, B3K 5A9
(902) 455-4286 nimbus.ca

Printed and bound in Canada
NB1690

Editor: Penelope Jackson
Cover Design: Heather Bryan
Interior Design: Brenda Jones & Heather Bryan

Library and Archives Canada Cataloguing in Publication

Title: Medicinal herbs of Western Canada : a pictorial manual / Brenda Jones.
Names: Jones, Brenda, 1953- author, illustrator.
Description: Includes index.
Identifiers: Canadiana (print) 2024028397X
Canadiana (ebook) 20240283988 | ISBN 9781774712658 (softcover)
ISBN 9781774712849 (EPUB)
Subjects: LCSH: Medicinal plants—Canada, Western—Identification.
LCSH: Medicinal plants—Canada, Western—Identification—Handbooks,
manuals, etc. | LCSH: Herbs—Therapeutic use—Canada, Western.
LCSH: Herbs—Therapeutic use—Canada, Western—Handbooks, manuals, etc. |
LCSH: Herbals—Canada, Western. | LCSH: Naturopathy. | LCSH: Botany,
Medical. | LCGFT: Field guides.
Classification: LCC QK99.C3 J665 2024 | DDC 581.6/3409712—dc23

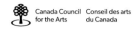 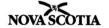

Nimbus Publishing acknowledges the financial support for its publishing activities from the Government of Canada, the Canada Council for the Arts, and from the Province of Nova Scotia. We are pleased to work in partnership with the Province of Nova Scotia to develop and promote our creative industries for the benefit of all Nova Scotians.

To all the intrepid wild crafters and nature lovers out there who thrive in the quiet nurturing energy of the fields, forests, and gardens throughout this country.

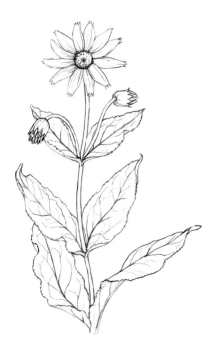

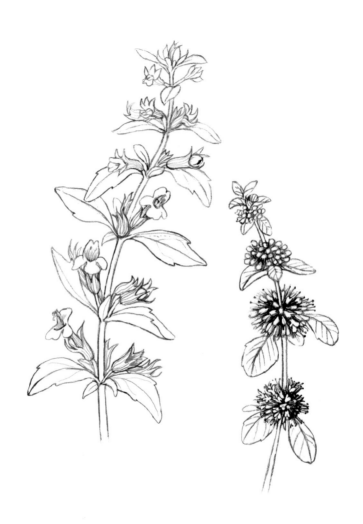

TABLE OF CONTENTS

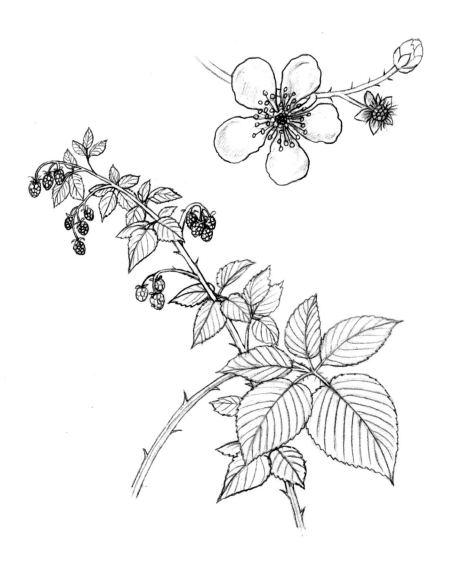

INTRODUCTION

Since ancient times, herbs have played a major role in healing in every culture around the world. Traditional remedies were passed down from one generation to another, using local plants and trees to cure disease, heal wounds, or ease pain. Particularly in Indigenous cultures, shamans, healers, and midwives played an important role in society, and their knowledge was gifted to future generations through word of mouth so as not to lose these important medicines. Unfortunately, over the last hundred years much of this knowledge has been lost due to the rise of modern science and the pharmaceutical industry, attempted genocide of many Indigenous cultures, and the destruction of rare species and their habitats. However, with the increase in chronic diseases and superbugs and the difficulties accessing healthcare in recent years, there has been a resurgence of interest in medicinal herbs as people attempt to find relief for themselves. Although drugs will always play a major role in the healthcare industry, they are not the only answer. There is room for a more gentle, holistic approach to healing and for working with nature and all the gifts the earth has given us.

Growing up on Prince Edward Island, I developed an interest in plants when I was very young. My mother and I would spend hours together in the woods and fields of our summer home, picking berries, hunting for wildflowers, and collecting specimens for a fairy garden. We would amass all sorts of mosses, Ground Spruce, Ghost Pipes, Tea Berries, Mayflowers, Violets and brightly coloured toadstools, arrange them in a tin pan with a few rocks and sticks, then set them up in the garden amongst the Hollyhocks to attract any magical creatures that might pass by. Although it was the time spent with my mother that I keep close to my heart, I also appreciate how she passed on her love of the forests and the flowers. Nature has been a source of grounding for me ever since, whether through planting my own garden and digging my fingers into the sweet-smelling soil, or just taking walks by myself in the countryside. There is healing energy in the earth, and the farther we are away from it, the more disconnected we are from our own spirit.

I think I only learned to truly appreciate the importance of that connection to the earth after spending thirty years in a big city. There came a point in my life where every cell in my body was trying to tell me to leave. I had a good job, friends, and family in the city, but my soul craved the water and the open fields and cool forests, where I could see the horizon and the stars and watch the sun rise and set and storms rolling in. By the time I reached my mid-fifties, I also had chronic digestive problems and insomnia and I was burnt out. I had to make a change.

That change came for me in the form of a small cottage on the East Coast where I could finally find silence, breathe, and immerse myself in Mother Nature. I soon developed a passion for the plants that grew wild in the surrounding fields, and over the next few years I began writing and illustrating pages and pages of information found in the stacks of books I had collected, to help me identify and remember all the different plants in my environment. When I discovered that many were medicinal and had a long history of use, I began experimenting with tinctures and teas and soon found ways of dealing with my own health issues. Before long I realized I was writing a book. Although I had spent my life illustrating children's books, *Medicinal Herbs of Eastern Canada* was the first one I created by myself.

When my publisher approached me to create another herb book, this time on western herbs, I was a bit skeptical. Living on the east coast, how could I possibly know what medicines are used in western Canada? To top it off, we were right in the middle of COVID-19 lockdowns across the country; I couldn't even travel. But I was pleased to have a project to keep me occupied while we were isolated for an undetermined amount of time, so I ordered as many books on western herbs that I could find, took some online courses, and went to work on the research.

At this point, since I started relatively late in life, I can't really call myself a true herbalist. I believe that title belongs to those who have dedicated their whole life to understanding herbs and using them to heal others. It takes many years of study and practice to understand how the body works, the subtle properties of each species of plant, and how they interact with patients on a deeply personal level. My real goal in creating these books was to provide a detailed illustration of each of the herbs available in the region to help people with identification, along with giving a clear description and ways the average person can become familiar with their properties and how to use them. I tried to include traditional uses as well as latest research on each of the herbs, using only the most reliable sources and databases available.

Some of the traditional remedies have not as yet been scientifically proven due to a lack of funding for research (they cannot be patented, so aren't seen as worth the money to research), but their use around the globe has been documented for centuries, so I'm confident that my information is accurate. However, we need to understand that we are complex creatures. What may work for one might not work for another. If you're faced with a serious health issue and looking for alternative treatments, be sure you consult a certified herbalist and discuss possible treatments and drug interactions with a healthcare professional. Comprehending the way the body and plant medicine work together, particularly when there are many complex issues, requires a keen intuition and self-knowledge that takes time to develop, but we are all capable of learning if our mind is uncluttered and our intention is clear.

Our society has become disconnected from nature over the last fifty years, especially with our device addiction that keeps us glued to a screen for the better part of our day. We depend on grocery stores for our food, and many children growing up in the city have no idea where our food comes from. Children are playing outside less, and opting to stay indoors with TV and video games instead. Is it any wonder people aren't comfortable in nature anymore?

However, since our experience of living through COVID-19, I have noticed a shift in perception of nature that gives me hope for future generations. Since contact with others outside of our immediate family was, for a couple of years, discouraged, more families were getting out on the trails, hiking and biking to relieve the boredom. Not surprisingly, they not only found that this activity made them feel better, but they also realized the fear they had of anything wild was completely unfounded. Research shows that immersion in nature is both pleasurable and highly beneficial to our health and well-being. It can lower blood pressure, reduce anxiety and stress, and even improve immunity to disease. I can only hope this book will encourage people to do more "forest bathing" and learn more about all the amazing plants on their journeys, what they can use for their own benefit, and what they need to avoid.

Since I began researching these books, I have started my own backyard garden, and now have dozens of edible and medicinal herbs, some of which I planted and some which have mysteriously appeared and made themselves at home over the years. Some are weeds that I welcome in and then regret as I watch them take over my yard, but all are tasty and nutritious. My salads over the summer months include many wildcrafted plants found either in my back-yard or within a thirty-mile radius: nutty-tasting Watercress, crunchy Purs-lane, Dandelion greens, Borage flowers, Violets, lemony Sorrel, spicy Mustard greens and Mint…and topped off with a few wild Strawberries.

It is important to note that if you are wildcrafting your herbs, you should be conscious of where you pick them and how abundant they are. Never use plants that grow along a busy highway or next to farmer's fields that are sprayed with pesticides or anywhere that might be contaminated. Always use plants that are healthy and strong, not eaten by insects or diseased, and make sure there are enough plants left behind that you won't be depleting the local population. Only take what you need, and if using the top of the plant, leave the roots intact so it can grow back. If there are only a few, or the species is endangered, leave them alone. I have gotten into the habit of leaving a pinch of tobacco when I take something from the environment; it reminds me that the plants are a gift and we should leave something in return. Indigenous Peoples have always been conscious of this, giving thanks for everything that is taken from the land; it is never taken for granted or wasted. We would all be better off learning from these teachings.

I should also emphasize the importance of correctly identifying any plant before consuming it. I have tried to include as much detail as possible to assist with identification because I want people to feel confident and comfortable using these plants. I have also included a section at the end of the book to help identify the most common poisonous plants, particularly the ones you should not touch. I urge you to consult it when gathering herbs or foraging in the wild, and to teach your children which ones to avoid. I can't stress enough that if you're not sure, do not eat it! There are many berries, not all included here, that might look tasty to a small child but may result in a nasty bellyache; they could even be deadly when consumed. Also be aware that a plant may be medicinal in small doses but could become toxic if not used properly, so please heed the warnings provided.

Spending time in the great outdoors can be so enriching, opening our minds and senses to the many gifts our natural world has to offer. When done with care and respect, it can teach us a great deal about ourselves.

Disclaimer

The information provided in this book is intended for educational purposes only. Every effort has been made to ensure the accuracy of this information through extensive research; however, I make no guarantees regarding errors or omissions and assume no legal responsibility for injuries resulting from the use of remedies in this book. The suggestions included are not intended as a substitute for professional medical care.

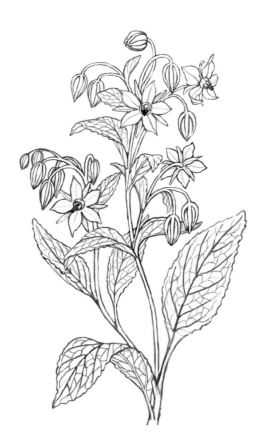

HERBAL PREPARATIONS

These are some of the most common methods of preparing herbs.

INTERNAL REMEDIES

| INFUSIONS |

Probably the simplest way of using herbs, infusions are simply teas made from a herb or a mixture of herbs in order to extract the healing properties. This method is best for the leafy parts and flowers of the plant, and they should be chopped fine to expose as much surface as possible. Since fresh herbs contain more water, we usually double the amount. A standard infusion consists of:
- 1 tsp. dried herbs or 2 tsp. fresh
- 1 cup boiling water
- Let infuse for 10–15 minutes, preferably in a covered teapot, particularly if the herb is fragrant, to retain the volatile oils. Strain into a cup and drink hot or cool.

| DECOCTIONS |

This method is used for more woody parts of the herb, like stems, bark, roots or rhizomes, and sometimes berries. They require a bit more steeping to extract the medicines and should be chopped as finely as possible before decocting. A standard decoction consists of:
- 1 tsp. to 1 tbsp. fresh or dried herbs, chopped or finely ground
- 1 cup cold water
- Place in a pot, cover, and heat on the stove until it comes to a boil. Reduce heat and simmer 20–40 minutes. Cool slightly and strain. You may make a larger batch, but leftovers should be refrigerated and used within 48 hours.

| TINCTURES |

Standard tinctures are made by macerating fresh or dried herbs in 40% alcohol, preferably vodka or brandy. (Other solvents like apple cider vinegar or glycerine may be used, but these are technically not tinctures). This method extracts more of the medicinal qualities and preserves them longer than if they were simply dried. The standard folk method for making alcohol tinctures is:

- For fresh herbs, fill a Mason jar about ⅔ full.
- For dried herbs, fill jar about ½ full.
- For roots, bark or berries, fill about ⅓ full.
- Make sure they are clean and dry, and chop or grind to increase surface exposure. Fill up the jar with alcohol. For a more precise measure, weigh the plant material so that there is a ratio of 1 part (in grams) to 2 parts alcohol (in millilitres) for fresh plants, and 1 part to 5 parts alcohol for dried plants.
- Cover and seal the jar. Check after a while to make sure the herbs are still covered, as some will expand and may spoil. Add more alcohol if necessary. Store in a cool, dry place for about 6 weeks, shaking the bottle periodically.
- After 6 weeks, strain the mixture into a measuring cup covered with several layers of cheesecloth. Gather up the cheesecloth with the plant material in it and squeeze out as much liquid as possible to get the maximum amount, as this is where it is more concentrated. Let settle and strain again if necessary. Pour through a funnel into an amber tincture bottle, label and date, and store in a dark cupboard.

NOTE: Some plants require a stronger alcohol in order to extract their medicines, particularly herbs containing resins, like cannabis or balsam. For these it's best to use pure, organic grain alcohol at 85–95%. Deviations from the standard tincture instructions are explained in the individual profiles.

| SYRUPS |

Syrups are a good way to make herbal concoctions more palatable, particularly if they happen to be strong and/or quite bitter. The sweetener, usually sugar or honey, also helps preserve the medicine for a longer period of time.
Here is a basic recipe for cough syrup:

- ⅓ cup dry herbs
- 2 cups cold water
- ½ cup honey or sugar
- Place woody herbs or roots and water in a saucepan and bring to a boil (if you have leaves or flowers, add them at the end of simmering time). Allow to simmer until liquid has reduced by about half. Cover the pan and let sit for an hour or so. Strain out plant matter and return the liquid to the pot. If adding honey, heat very gently, just enough to soften the honey, and remove from heat. If sugar is added, heat just long enough to dissolve the sugar. If you wish, you can add up to 3 tbsp. of brandy or other alcohol.

| INFUSED OILS |

Herbs can easily be infused into oils for use as massage oil, to relieve itchiness, soreness, or inflammation, as a bath oil, or for culinary use. We typically use organic cold-pressed virgin olive oil, but sweet almond, grapeseed, jojoba, or coconut oils can also be used. They will last up to a year if kept in a cool, dark place.

Make sure herbs are clean and dry. If using fresh herbs, do not wash them, as you want the least amount of moisture possible in the jar. Leave on the counter for a couple of days to let bugs escape and any moisture to evaporate, then chop and pack into a sterilized Mason jar, up to ¾ full. I prefer to use dried herbs as they are less likely to spoil.

Cover with oil, leaving ½ inch at the top and making sure that plant material is completely submerged. Use a knife to release any air bubbles in the liquid. Cover with wax paper and screw on lid. Leave in a dark place for 4–6 weeks, shaking occasionally.

Strain into a bowl covered with cheesecloth and squeeze out as much liquid as possible. If you used fresh herbs, check after a few hours to see if any water has settled to the bottom before pouring into the bottle as you'll want to leave it behind. Using a funnel, pour oil into a clean, dry, sterilized bottle and label.

| OINTMENTS AND SALVES |

These are a great way to protect and soothe inflamed skin and to heal sores and wounds. They contain oils or fats but no water, so they form a layer on top of the skin rather than sinking into it like a cream. Any kind of infused oil may be used in this basic recipe.
- 20 grams beeswax
- 100 ml. herb-infused oil
- 1 small (120 ml.) Mason jar, sterilized
- Gently warm the beeswax and oil together in a double boiler or Pyrex bowl set into a pan of water. When wax has melted, place a drop on a saucer and place in the freezer for a minute to test the consistency. If it's too hard, add a little more oil, if too soft, add more beeswax. Remove from heat, cool slightly and add a few drops of essential oil if desired.

| LINIMENTS |

A liniment is basically a mixture of a strong herbal decoction and alcohol, which is readily absorbed into the skin to relieve the pain of sprains, sore muscles, or broken bones. The addition of alcohol adds to the shelf life of the decoction and aids absorption of the herbs. Here is a basic recipe:
- 1 part vodka or rubbing alcohol

- 2 parts decoction (should be well strained before adding alcohol)
- You can also make a good liniment by placing a mixture of herbs in a steril-ized jar and adding enough Witch Hazel or rubbing alcohol to cover. Screw on lid and let the mixture sit for 4–8 weeks. Strain and pour into a sterilized bottle or spray bottle and label to remind you that it is NOT to be taken internally. It will keep for about a year.

EXTERNAL REMEDIES

| POULTICES |

A poultice consists of solid fresh plant material that has been mashed or bruised to release the medicines, or dried herbs that have been ground and made into a paste by adding warm water. This paste is placed directly on to the skin and can be covered with a hot water bottle if desired. They are usually made from warming and stimulating herbs, vulneraries, astringents, or emollients.

| COMPRESSES |

Compresses or fomentations are clean cloths like gauze or cotton which have been soaked in a hot infusion or decoction. They are placed on the affected area and kept as hot as possible to enhance the action of the herbs. A hot water bottle can be placed on top of the compress to keep it warm for a longer period of time. Vulnerary herbs, stimulants, and diaphoretics make good compresses.

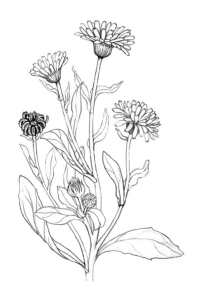

ALFALFA

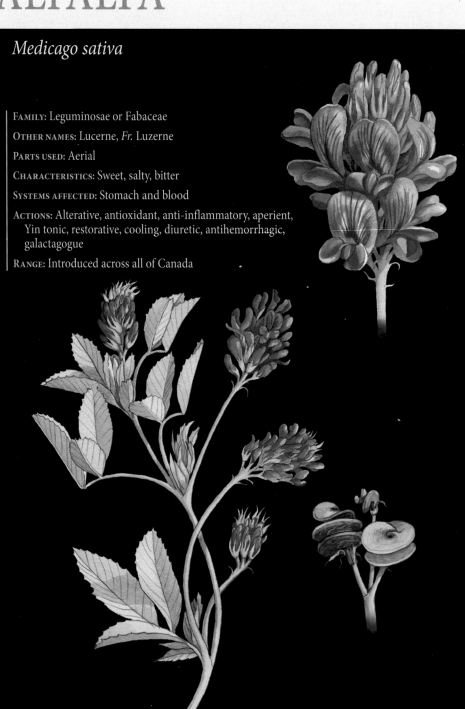

Medicago sativa

FAMILY: Leguminosae or Fabaceae

OTHER NAMES: Lucerne, *Fr.* Luzerne

PARTS USED: Aerial

CHARACTERISTICS: Sweet, salty, bitter

SYSTEMS AFFECTED: Stomach and blood

ACTIONS: Alterative, antioxidant, anti-inflammatory, aperient, Yin tonic, restorative, cooling, diuretic, antihemorrhagic, galactagogue

RANGE: Introduced across all of Canada

This colourful perennial has been cultivated as a forage crop for hundreds of years. At full size it may reach a height of up to 1 metre. It somewhat resembles Clover, but its leaves grow more elongated as it matures and are notched at the tips. The flowers that appear in June or July range from pink to mauve or purple and are pollinated by bees or butterflies. Grown for fodder, it also increases milk production in livestock and fertilizes the fields, its long roots fixing nitrogen in the soil after a couple of years of growth, making it one of nature's best green manures. It grows in sunny locations and well-drained soil and can be picked during the summer and dried for later use.

MEDICINAL USES:

Wasting diseases, lack of appetite, anemia, hemorrhage, cystitis

- Leaves and young shoots are edible, raw or cooked. Very nutritious, rich in chlorophyll, vitamins A, B, C, K, protein, and minerals.
- Restorative tonic, helps build weight and improve digestion during convalescence, warms the stomach, increases appetite, restores strength and vitality. Tonic for the weak and emaciated, where there is poor assimilation of nutrients, despondency, and chronic indigestion. Good for peptic ulcers and slow peristalsis.
- Relieves chronic and acute urinary tract infections, with backache and sparse urination. Diuretic, helps with prostate irritations.
- Nourishes the blood, helps anemia, slows hemorrhaging. Estrogenic properties help ease menopausal symptoms and PMS. Increases milk production in lactating women. May help lower cholesterol.
- Works slowly and penetrates deep into the body where chronic problems originate. Should be taken regularly over long periods to correct chronic problems.

OTHER USES:
- Young shoots, flowers, and sprouts are good in salads.
- A yellow dye can be made from the seeds.
- Fibre from the plant has been used to make paper.

INFUSION: 1–2 tsp. dried herb in 1 cup of boiling water. Infuse 5–10 minutes. Drink 3 times a day.

TINCTURE: 1 ml. 2–3 times daily.

COMBINATIONS:

May be combined with Nettles for use as a blood tonic, Red Clover as a nutritive tonic, or add Ginseng and Ashwagandha for anemia.

CAUTION: Contains saponin-like substances. Do not eat in large quantities. Avoid during pregnancy, and with hormone-sensitive cancers. May trigger attacks in people with systemic lupus erythematosus; avoid in autoimmune diseases and gout. Seeds should not be eaten, as they contain canavanine, a toxic amino acid. Avoid use if taking Warfarin.

AMERICAN ASPEN

Populus tremuloides

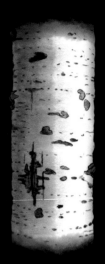

FAMILY: Salicaceae

OTHER NAMES: Quaking Aspen, Trembling Aspen, Poplar, *Fr.* Peuplier faux-tremble

PARTS USED: Inner bark, root, leaf buds

CHARACTERISTICS: Bitter, astringent

SYSTEMS AFFECTED: Digestive, urinary, reproductive

ACTIONS: Antimicrobial, analgesic, anti-inflammatory, astringent, diuretic, diaphoretic, febrifuge, nervine, vermifuge, antiscorbutic, expectorant, purgative

RANGE: Native across all of Canada

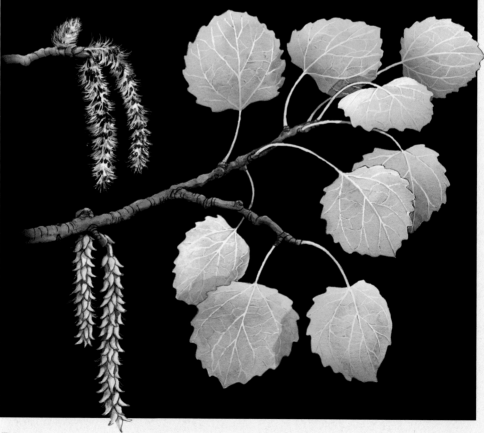

Quaking or American Aspen has been so-named because of the gentle rustling noise made by its leaves in even the slightest of breezes. It's a native deciduous tree from the Willow family found across Canada, usually under 15 metres tall, and, like the Willow, has been used for centuries for its pain-relieving properties. Short-lived and fast-growing, it is dioecious, meaning male catkins (grey and fuzzy) and female catkins (green and smooth) grow on separate trees. Leaves are alternate and oval or heart-shaped, shiny green on top and dull or silvery underneath, turning yellow-orange in the fall, with rounded teeth. The bark of younger trees is creamy white, grey, or greenish white with dark markings and covered in a powdery coating, where older bark is dark grey to greenish brown, rough and furrowed. The trees multiply by sending out rhizomes, forming large groves. Bark should be taken from lateral branches so as not to weaken the tree. Peel off the outer bark and dry for later use.

MEDICINAL USES:

Pain, digestive and liver disorders, menstrual cramps and excessive bleeding, urinary infection, anorexia, arthritis, wounds

- Dried inner bark contains salicin, from which aspirin is derived. Decoction or massage oil made from the bark relieves pain and inflammation from arthritis, rheumatism, fibromyalgia, gout, lower back pain.
- Relieves digestive disturbances due to sluggishness and liver disorders, tonifies the digestive tract. Relieves chronic diarrhea and stimulates bile production.
- Appetite stimulant, it may help with anorexia and relieve stomach pain.
- Decoction from root bark taken to relieve cramps, excessive menstrual bleeding, leukorrhea.
- Warm tea can be taken for fevers, colds, or coughs, and gargled for sore throat.
- Anti-inflammatory and antiseptic properties help with cystitis.
- Light powder on bark used to stop bleeding, prevent hair growth, and mixed with jojoba oil can be used as sunscreen.
- Bark or leaf may be chewed and packed around a tooth to relieve toothache.
- Poultice from mashed bark or root relieves hemorrhoids, skin inflammation, rashes, wounds, burns.

OTHER USES:
- Inner bark is sweet and edible raw or added to soups. The inner bark can be ground and added to flour for bread. Catkins also edible and high in Vitamin C, but bitter.
- Sap may be tapped and drunk as a beverage.
- Long shoots used in basket-making.

DECOCTION: Simmer 1 tsp. dried bark in 1¼ cups water for 10–15 minutes. Let steep for 1 hour, take ¼–½ cup up to 4 times a day.

TINCTURE: 1 part dry bark to 2 parts vodka/distilled water mix (1:1). Take 15–20 drops before meals to aid digestion, 1–10 drops to relieve anxiety.

COMBINATIONS:

Combine with uva-ursi (Bearberry) to make an excellent tonic for bladder infections.

CAUTION: Avoid use internally if sensitive to aspirin.

AMERICAN BUGLEWEED

Lycopus americanus
L. uniflorus

FAMILY: Lamiaceae

OTHER NAMES: *L. americanus*: American Water-horehound, Cut-leaved Bugleweed, *Fr.* Lycope d'Amérique; *L. uniflorus*: Northern Bugleweed, *Fr.* Lycope uniflore

PARTS USED: Whole plant

CHARACTERISTICS: Bitter, cooling, drying

SYSTEMS AFFECTED: Lungs, heart, thyroid

ACTIONS: Anti-inflammatory, antitussive, astringent, cardiac tonic, mildly narcotic, sedative

RANGE: Native across all provinces except Labrador

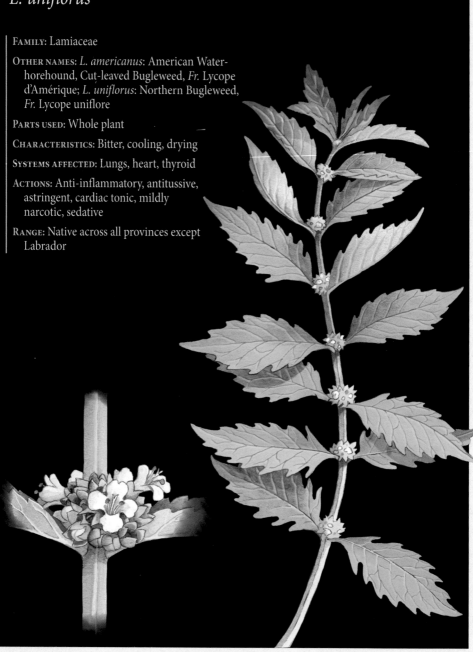

This native perennial is a member of the mint family and would easily be confused with mint if not for the lack of the distinctive aroma. *L. americanus* and *L. uniflorus* are quite similar and are interchangeable medicinally, along with another European relative, *L. europaeus*. They should not be confused with a plant which is often called Bugleweed or Common Bugle, *Ajuga reptans*, which belongs to another family of herbs. *Lycopus americanus* grows up to a height of around 60 cm. Its usually unbranched stem is sometimes covered in fine hairs and is squarish with opposite, lance-shaped, hairless leaves that are narrowly lobed towards the base but more coarsely toothed at the top. Often the central vein has fine hairs on the underside. The tiny flowers grow in clusters in the leaf axils, the calyx forming a tube with 4 broad teeth. The flower is also in form of a tube with 4 fused petals and may be white or pinkish with tiny pink spots, replaced by 4 small square-shaped nutlets in late summer. Usually found in low, wet places, the whole plant can be gathered during the summer and dried for future use.

MEDICINAL USES:

Hyperactive thyroid, Graves' disease, tachycardia, anxiety, coughs, pulmonary bleeding

- Studies show promise in the treatment of hyperthyroid disorders and Graves' disease. Contains rosmarinic acid, which calms the activity of thyroid-stimulating hormone, or TSH. Reduces elevated heart rate common in hyperthyroidism, as well as high blood pressure and hyperthermia. Often combined with Lemon Balm and Motherwort.
- Useful for a dry, irritable cough with heat, inflammation, and a frequent and small amount of bleeding from the lungs, especially in chronic bronchitis and passive pulmonary hemorrhage (often combined with Wild Cherry, Pleurisy Root, Trillium, and Yarrow).
- Mild sedative. Traditionally used by Cherokee people to calm the heart and promote sleep by chewing the roots, and to treat snake bites by chewing the root and swallowing half, applying the rest to the wound. Often fed to children to give "eloquence of speech."
- Heart tonic, where there is tachycardia or rapid heartbeat with weak circulation. Slows and strengthens the heart, reduces inflammation and relieves anxiety and insomnia, particularly when recovering from debilitating diseases where heartbeat affects the sleep.
- Mild gastric tonic, improves digestion, calms upset stomach.
- Eases excessive menstrual bleeding.

TINCTURE: Fresh 1:2 in 50% alcohol. Take 10–30 drops up to 4 times a day.

INFUSION: 2 tbsp. to 2 cups of boiling water. Take 1 cup 3 times a day.

CAUTION: Plant generally considered safe, except for hypothyroid conditions. May reduce blood sugar, so use with caution if you have diabetes. Not advised during pregnancy as there have been no studies to verify safety.

ARROWLEAF BALSAMROOT

Balsamorhiza sagittata

FAMILY: Asteraceae

OTHER NAMES: Oregon Sunflower, Breadroot, *Fr.* Balsamorhize à feuilles sagittées

PARTS USED: Whole plant

CHARACTERISTICS: Pungent, warm, dry

SYSTEMS AFFECTED: Stomach and lungs

ACTIONS: Antirheumatic, antimicrobial, diuretic, diaphoretic, febrifuge, vulnerary

RANGE: Native to southern British Columbia, Alberta, and Saskatchewan

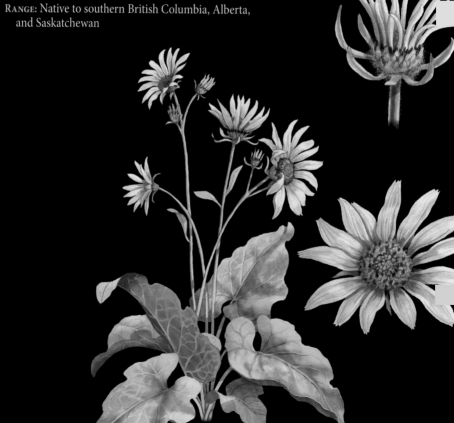

One of the most important plants for Indigenous Peoples of British Columbia, this large perennial was once a major food source, its long taproot, young shoots, and seeds providing nourishment and medicine throughout the year. Growing on rocky hillsides and grasslands, the woody root of these plants may reach 1.5–2.4 metres deep as they get older, is pungent and resinous in taste, and is usually the part used in making medicines. Several leaf stems arise from the hairy crown; the soft basal leaves are heart-shaped, pointed at the tip, and often up to 60 cm. long. Other small lance-shaped leaves grow on the flower stems, which are 15–81 cm. and topped with one or several yellow sunflower-like blooms. The whole plant smells resinous when rubbed. It provides food and shelter to wildlife and is of great benefit to the environment, the long roots holding soil together and preventing erosion. Harvest roots when they're about the size of a large carrot, as they are easier to break apart. Use a hatchet or machete to chop them up into small pieces for tincturing.

MEDICINAL USES:

Stomach problems, colds, fevers, lung congestion, sore throat, skin irritations

- Used widely by Indigenous Peoples, mostly for stomach complaints and toothaches.
- Infusion or tincture of the whole plant is used for stomach pains, colds, coughs, fevers, and headaches. It promotes the flow of mucous in the respiratory tract, releases mucous in the sinuses, and soothes inflammation. Its mild antimicrobial activity stimulates white blood cells and aids the immune system to fight infection.
- Root may be chewed for sore throat, mouth sores or toothaches. A syrup of the roots soothes coughs and sore throat.
- A decoction of the root is used at the onset of labour to ease pains and delivery.
- The root or leaves can be pounded to use as a poultice on wounds, burns, blisters, bites, swellings, or sores. Infused oil eases pain of rheumatism.
- A few drops of tincture may relieve Seasonal Affective Disorder (SAD) and lift the spirits.

OTHER USES:
- Young shoots can be eaten raw or steamed; flower stems and young leaf stalks eaten raw or cooked. Traditionally, the root was usually roasted for several days in fire pits to make it sweeter and more digestible.
- The seeds can be dried and roasted and pounded into a meal.
- An infusion of the root was sometimes used to promote hair growth.

TINCTURE: 1 part dried root to 5 parts alcohol (65%). Take 15–50 drops up to 4 times a day in hot water. May be combined with Elderberry or Cottonwood bud tincture and honey for colds and sore throat.

CAUTION: May cause kidney irritation in large doses, but generally the whole plant is safe to use.

BALSAM POPLAR, BLACK COTTONWOOD

Populus balsamifera (Balsam Poplar)
ssp. P. trichocarpa (Black Cottonwood)

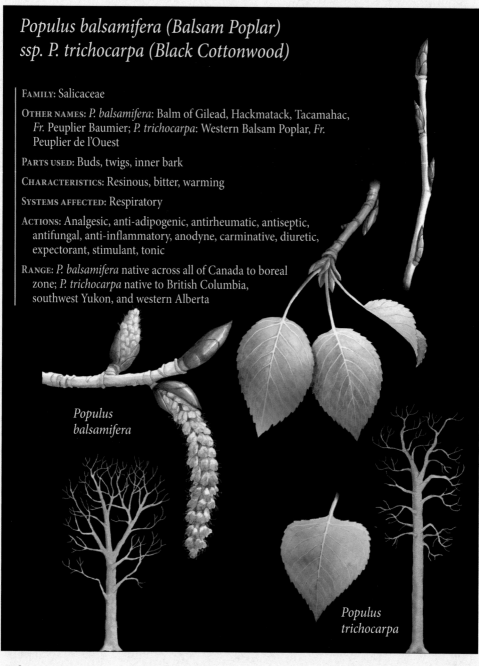

FAMILY: Salicaceae

OTHER NAMES: *P. balsamifera*: Balm of Gilead, Hackmatack, Tacamahac, *Fr.* Peuplier Baumier; *P. trichocarpa*: Western Balsam Poplar, *Fr.* Peuplier de l'Ouest

PARTS USED: Buds, twigs, inner bark

CHARACTERISTICS: Resinous, bitter, warming

SYSTEMS AFFECTED: Respiratory

ACTIONS: Analgesic, anti-adipogenic, antirheumatic, antiseptic, antifungal, anti-inflammatory, anodyne, carminative, diuretic, expectorant, stimulant, tonic

RANGE: *P. balsamifera* native across all of Canada to boreal zone; *P. trichocarpa* native to British Columbia, southwest Yukon, and western Alberta

Populus balsamifera

Populus trichocarpa

These native deciduous trees from the Willow family are very highly valued by many Indigenous Peoples across North America. Balsam Poplar and Black Cottonwood are usually found near damp areas and have very similar properties and uses, but only the latter grows exclusively in temperate climates of western Canada and the US, and tends to be quite a bit taller, often up to 35 metres. The resinous, fragrant leaf buds are the parts most used for medicine and are usually gathered in late winter or early spring. The leaves that emerge in spring are dark green on top, light blue-grey underneath, ovate, and finely serrated, the Black Cottonwood leaf tending to be flatter at the base. Flowers are either male or female, and only one sex is found on a single tree. In the spring, they emerge as greenish or reddish catkins, which then produce globular fruit that split open, turning to a cottony fluff that blows off in the wind, spreading the seeds. Harvest buds early, preferably from fallen branches, as the buds are larger higher up on the tree and it's a more sustainable way to collect them. Inner bark can be taken from these branches as well, and twigs may simply be chopped into smaller pieces.

MEDICINAL USES:

Upper respiratory tract infections, fevers, skin problems, rheumatism, muscle pain

- Resin from the buds can stimulate lungs to expel mucous and heal infection, particularly in cases of dry asthma and when cough is longstanding and unproductive.
- Buds and inner bark contain salicin, from which aspirin is derived, helping to reduce fevers and pain from sore muscles, rheumatism, or menstrual pain.
- Oil made from the bud resin can be used as is or in a salve for mild burns or sunburn, to soothe skin inflammation, disinfect, and ease the pain of arthritic joints, sprains, carpal tunnel, and sore muscles. New research suggests it may be effective in treating psoriasis. It reduces swelling and inflammation and prevents infection. Oil and salve will last for many years due to natural preservatives.
- Inner bark is anti-inflammatory and anodyne. It can be eaten fresh off the tree or dried and ground to use as a thickener for soups or added to bread.
- A few drops of tincture in water aids digestion, can be gargled for sore throats, or to heal mouth or gum infections.

OTHER USES:
- An extract made from the shoots can be used as a rooting hormone for cuttings. Soak the shoots in cold water for 24 hours.
- Infuse the buds in cream, then whip the cream for a delicious treat with a caramel-like flavour.
- Indigenous Peoples have traditionally used the resin to waterproof the seams of canoes or burned it to repel mosquitoes.

TINCTURE: Pack a Mason jar ¼ full with fresh buds, fill jar with alcohol (at least 75%), allow it to sit for 4–6 weeks, shaking often. Strain and bottle. Use diluted in water, 15–30 drops up to 4 times a day.

OIL: Put 1 cup fresh buds into a quart Mason jar, fill with olive oil. Cover and keep in a warm place for 4–6 weeks. Strain and bottle. Use as a chest rub for respiratory infections, sprains, sore muscles, arthritis. May be combined with St. John's Wort and/or Wild Bergamot oil for burns.

CAUTION: Avoid use internally if sensitive to aspirin. It is recommended to wear gloves while gathering the buds as the resin can be difficult to remove once it coats your hands.

BEARBERRY

Arctostaphylos uva-ursi

FAMILY: Ericaceae

OTHER NAMES: Mealberry, Foxberry, Hog Cranberry, Kinnikinnick,
Fr. Raisin d'ours

PARTS USED: Leaves, stems, fruit

CHARACTERISTICS: Bitter, astringent, cool

SYSTEMS AFFECTED: Heart, kidney, bladder, small intestine, liver

ACTIONS: Anti-inflammatory, antiseptic, astringent, diuretic,
urinary antiseptic, tonic

RANGE: Native across all of Canada

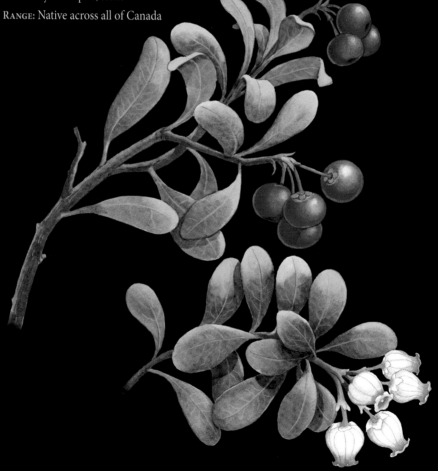

This low-growing evergreen shrub probably earned its name, *uva-ursi*, which means "bear's grape," from the fact that bears tend to find the berries tasty—whereas people consider the flavour unpleasant. Growing to a height of about 20 cm., its trailing branches are short and woody, covered in a pale brown bark. The shoots are slightly hairy and rise upward from the stems. The leaves are leathery and spoon-shaped, dark green on top and paler underneath with a coarse network of veins. The flowers appear in drooping clusters in June, each one urn-shaped, usually white, sometimes with a reddish lip. Berries appear in the fall and resemble a small red currant. It grows in dry open woods, in gravelly or sandy soils. Collect leaves in September or October, only in fine, dry weather when the dew has evaporated, taking only green, unblemished leaves. Dry in the sun if possible; if not, use a warm, dry, well-ventilated shed.

MEDICINAL USES:

Cystitis, headaches, wounds, general tonic

- This herb contains the effective anti-inflammatory and antiseptic components hydroquinone, arbutin, and methyl arbutin, making *uva-ursi* a natural diuretic and a traditional treatment for bladder and urinary tract infections for hundreds of years. It is also a powerful astringent, soothing and tonifying the entire urinary system. The leaves contain a recognized antibacterial that works best if the patient is on a vegetable-based diet where the urine is alkaline. Works to relieve cystitis, urethritis, kidney and bladder stones, and other inflammatory diseases of the urinary tract.
- Has been used in folk medicine for years as a headache remedy. The leaves are dried and smoked, producing a mild narcotic effect.
- Salve made from the fruit can speed healing when applied to wounds.
- Traditionally used to treat leukorrhea and chronic diarrhea.

OTHER USES: Contains tannins, which have been used for tanning leather.

INFUSION: For urinary tract infection, put 1 tsp. dried leaves into 1 cup boiling water. Steep for 10–15 minutes, then sip slowly for 3 or 4 hours or until symptoms subside. Don't exceed ¼ cup at a time, to avoid stomach upset. May be continued for several days afterward to prevent recurrence.

COMBINATIONS:

May be used with Corn silk, Marshmallow root, Echinacea, and Licorice root in formulas for urinary tract infections.

CAUTION: May cause nausea or constipation if taken in large quantities. Prolonged use may cause stomach and liver problems. Use only under the care of a professional if you're pregnant or nursing. Do not give to children.

BLACKBERRY

Rubus allegheniensis (Allegheny Blackberry)
R. armeniacus (Himalayan Blackberry)
R. ursinus (Trailing Blackberry)

FAMILY: Rosaceae

OTHER NAMES: *Fr.* Mûrier

PARTS USED: Leaves, fruit, root bark

CHARACTERISTICS: Berries sweet, leaves and root bark astringent, cool

SYSTEMS AFFECTED: Upper and lower GI tract, urinary

ACTIONS: Astringent, antiseptic, antioxidant, anti-inflammatory, diuretic, tonic

RANGE: *R. allegheniensis* introduced in British Columbia, native southern Ontario to Maritimes; *R. armeniacus* introduced in British Columbia, Manitoba to Maritimes; *R. ursinus* native to southern British Columbia

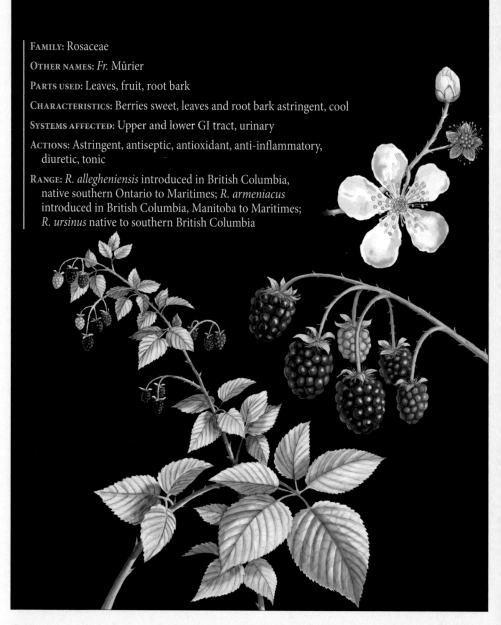

Many different varieties of Blackberry grow throughout Canada, their invasive nature, along with thorns and prickles, annoying those who are oblivious to their many attributes. Like its European cousin *R. fruticosus*, it is a perennial shrub composed of arching reddish stems and can grow from 2 to 5 metres tall, depending on the species. Its toothed compound leaves grow in groups of 3 or 5 arranged alternately up the stem. Clusters of white or pinkish 5-petalled flowers appear in early summer and turn into green fruit in August as the flowers die back. These ripen to red, and then turn dark purple or black as they become succulent, sweet, juicy berries that can be eaten by the handful. You can tell the difference between raspberries and blackberries by the core: a raspberry's core is hollow, whereas a blackberry's core is solid when picked. The leaves can be harvested during flowering and thoroughly dried for later use; the roots may be dug up at any time, the bark peeled off and dried in the oven. Pay special attention to where you harvest Trailing Blackberry, avoiding slash and burn piles as diesel residue may be present. Observe spraying notices and avoid plants with disfigured leaves or flowers as this may indicate contamination. Also, be aware that black bears love these berries and may be present.

MEDICINAL USES:

Diarrhea, urinary tract infections, mouth infections, bleeding, hemorrhoids

- Leaves and root bark contain tannins, which are astringent and help dry and tighten tissues, resolve mucous, and control bleeding. Can resolve diarrhea and dysentery, especially in children. Reduces inflammation in the intestinal tract, relieves hemorrhoids. Root contains higher concentrations.
- Infusion of leaves or decoction of root bark makes a good mouthwash for spongy gums, thrush, mouth ulcers, toothaches.
- Leaves and root bark, along with juice of the berries, have traditionally been used to treat anemia, menorrhagia, and leukorrhea. Leaf extract has been shown to have hypoglycemic properties.
- Poultice can stop minor bleeding and help heal skin ulcers, bruises, psoriasis.
- Decoction of root bark is diuretic and helps with urinary problems.
- Berries are highly nutritious, containing vitamins C and K, manganese, and fibre. They are known for their anticancerous properties, as they are rich in antioxidants that destroy free radicals and strengthen immunity.

OTHER USES: Plump berries make a tasty jam, especially when mixed with blackcurrants. May be used to make wine or added to brandy or other sweetened alcohol to make liqueurs.

INFUSION: 2 tbsp. dried leaves in 2 cups of water. Cool and drink ½ cup every couple of hours for diarrhea.

DECOCTION: 1 ounce of root bark boiled in 3½ cups water. Reduce to 2½ cups. Take ½ cup every 2 hours.

CAUTION: Wilted leaves may be toxic. Use either fresh or fully dried. Use in moderation.

BLUE COHOSH

Caulophyllum thalictroides

FAMILY: Berberidaceae

OTHER NAMES: Papoose Root, Blueberry Root, *Fr.* Cohosh Bleu, Léontice faux-pigamon

PARTS USED: Root, rhizome

CHARACTERISTICS: Warming, relaxing, drying, acrid, bitter

SYSTEMS AFFECTED: Liver

ACTIONS: Antispasmodic, anti-inflammatory, emmenagogue, relaxing nervine, uterine tonic, abortifacient

RANGE: Native from Manitoba to Nova Scotia

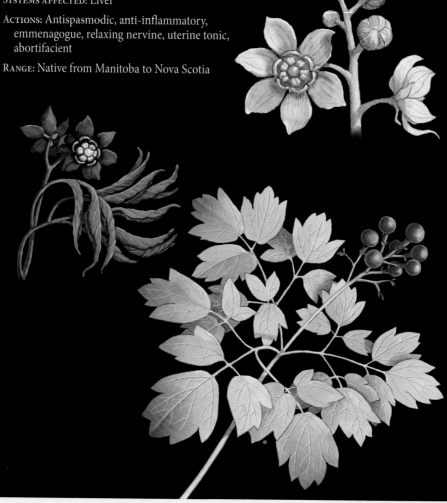

Blue Cohosh is another herb traditionally labelled as a women's herb, as it was historically used by Indigenous Peoples and settlers for menstrual problems and during childbirth. The erect central stem of this woodland perennial grows from 30 cm. to 90 cm. tall, is smooth and light green to purplish in colour, and terminates in a panicle of small flowers with 6 sepals that are greenish yellow or purplish, with insignificant yellow-green petals, 6 yellow stamens, and a round beak-like ovary. It blooms from mid to late spring before the leaves have fully developed, then the flowers are replaced by round green berries which eventually turn bright blue later in the summer. Roots should be collected in the fall and dried for later use in teas or tinctures. The berries and aerial parts are usually considered to be toxic.

MEDICINAL USES:

Childbirth, delayed menstruation, cramps, rheumatism, spasmodic coughing, anxiety

- Contains several active alkaloids and saponins which have been proven to act on uterine muscles, resulting in an oxytocic response, increasing the strength of uterine contractions. Often used by midwives to prepare a woman for childbirth in a formula called "Mother's Cordial," containing Partridge Berry, Raspberry Leaf, Black Cohosh, and False Unicorn. It eases pain and strengthens contractions. Particularly useful if labour is slow and the mother is exhausted. Should only be used under supervision and in small doses.
- Contains caulosaponin, which encourages menstruation. Uterine tonic, for inflammation, cramps, delayed menstruation, dysmenorrhea, breast pain, leukorrhea, vaginitis.
- Can ease arthritis and rheumatic pain, neuralgia.
- May help with spasmodic asthma, whooping cough, bronchitis.
- In formulas for anxiety, often combined with Skullcap.
- Used externally for toothache and as a remedy for Poison Oak or Poison Ivy.

OTHER USES: Some claim the seeds can be roasted to use as a coffee substitute (the roasting process is supposed to remove the toxins). However, it is not recommended.

TINCTURE: 1:5 in 60% alcohol. Take 5 drops every 4 hours or as advised by a professional. Best if used in formulas.

CAUTION: Use only root, as aerial parts may be toxic. Not for use during pregnancy prior to labour or if trying to get pregnant, as it provokes uterine contractions and may cause a miscarriage. Excessive doses may cause high blood pressure, nausea, vomiting, incoordination. Contraindicated for people with angina, high blood pressure, or heart disease, as it may cause narrowing of blood vessels to the heart. Avoid in hyperglycemia as it raises blood sugar levels. Powdered root may cause irritation of the mucous membranes. Touching plant may cause irritation in some people. Use only under strict supervision by a herbal practitioner.

BLUE ELDER

Sambucus cerulea or Sambucus nigra ssp. cerulea
S. canadensis (Common Elderberry)

FAMILY: Caprifoliaceae

OTHER NAMES: Blueberry Elder, American Elder, *Fr.* Sureau bleu

PARTS USED: Flowers, berries, leaves

CHARACTERISTICS: Acrid, bitter, cool. Flowers: sweet, cool, drying

SYSTEMS AFFECTED: Lungs, liver

ACTIONS: Flowers are diaphoretic, anti-catarrhal, mildly sedative; berries are diaphoretic, diuretic, laxative, antioxidant; leaves are emollient, vulnerary, purgative, expectorant, diuretic

RANGE: *S. cerulea* native to British Columbia; *S. canadensis* native from Manitoba to Maritimes

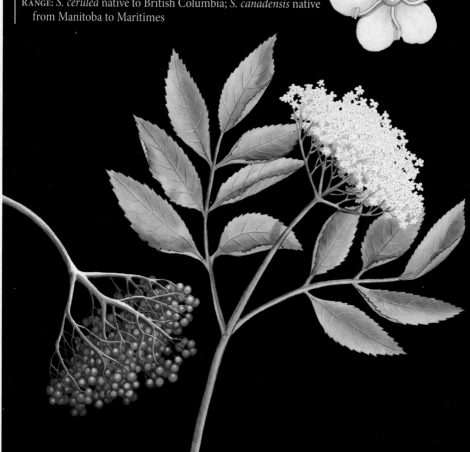

Sambucus cerulea is an indigenous shrub that very closely resembles its black European (*S. nigra*) and North American (*S. canadensis*) relatives both in appearance and medicinal properties. It grows to a height of up to 4 metres, with paired opposite leaves and one extra at the end of each branch, each finely serrated, oval, and pointed. The whitish flowers appear in July, growing in many large umbels and having a somewhat peculiar aroma. They develop into blue berries in the fall, which are covered in a white coating, making them look light blue or grey. They should only be used when completely ripe. The young branches contain a soft pith that is easily removed and was once used to make pipes or musical instruments; however, the fresh stems are poisonous and should be aged at least a year. Flowers should be harvested gently and dried quickly in a cool oven or on a screen. The berries may be gathered in the fall and dried or frozen immediately for later use. They should not be consumed raw. Store in an airtight container.

MEDICINAL USES:
Colds, flu, sinusitis, skin ailments

* Berries are nutritious, rich in antioxidants, flavonoids, vitamins, and minerals.
* Useful in first stages of cold or flu, upper respiratory tract infection, sinusitis, hay fever. Elder flower tea promotes expectoration and perspiration and can be taken hot before going to bed. It can be mixed with peppermint if desired. Syrup of the berries (below) has been proven to reduce symptoms and duration of colds and flu if taken at the first sign.
* Flowers and leaves are used in ointments and lotions to treat burns, rashes, bruises, sprains, and minor skin ailments, and to diminish wrinkles.
* Tea made from the flowers is a mild laxative and diuretic, and warm compresses may reduce pain of rheumatism, arthritis, and inflamed swellings. A cold infusion is said to be effective in relief of swollen glands and scrofula.
* Strained Elder flower tea that has been cooled with ¼ tsp. salt added per cup makes a good eyewash for inflammations.
* Elder berry wine was once used to ease arthritic pains.

FOLKLORE: There are many myths surrounding this bush that date far back and span across many cultures. Medieval beliefs held it to be a symbol of death and bad luck. In Northern Europe it was believed a dryad, Hylde Moer, lived in the tree, and if it was cut or used for furniture she would haunt the ones responsible. In England in the seventeenth century it was thought the tree would provide protection against witches and a twig was carried in the pocket to prevent rheumatism.

INFUSION FOR FLU WITH FEVER: Equal parts Elder flower, Yarrow, and Peppermint to make 2 tbsp. in 1 cup of boiling water (3 or 4 slices of Ginger may also be added). Take a warm bath and drink hot before bed. Infusions are best consumed within 12–24 hours (after this time, a bitter taste can emerge.)

ELDERBERRY SYRUP: Put ripe, dried, or frozen berries in a pot, add enough water just to cover, a few slices of fresh Ginger, and a couple of Cloves. Simmer over low heat, mashing until mushy and liquid is reduced by half. Strain through a sieve into a measuring cup, adding up to the same amount of unpasteurized honey to the juice, along with a pinch of Cinnamon and a squirt of Lemon juice to taste. Reheat gently just enough to melt the honey, add some brandy if desired (helps to preserve it; there should be a ratio of 20% alcohol to 80% syrup). Store in refrigerator. Take 1 tbsp. every hour at onset of a cold or flu, then 3 or 4 tbsp. per day till symptoms improve.

CAUTION: Do not use stems or leaves in infusions, only flowers. Stems are considered mildly poisonous. Raw berries may cause nausea, dizziness, or diarrhea in some people. Do not use berries from Red Elder as they are toxic. Use gloves when handling as some people may be sensitive to the sap.

BLUE VERVAIN

Verbena hastata

FAMILY: Verbenaceae

OTHER NAMES: Blue Verbena, Indian Hyssop, Swamp Verbena, Herba Sacra, *Fr.* Verveine bleue

PARTS USED: Whole plant

CHARACTERISTICS: Cold, bitter, drying; root astringent

SYSTEMS AFFECTED: Liver/gallbladder, spleen, nervous system, digestive, cardiovascular, urinary

ACTIONS: Astringent, anticatarrhal, antispasmodic, bitter tonic, diaphoretic, diuretic, expectorant, emmenagogue, emetic (in large doses), nervine, febrifuge, galactagogue, vulnerary, tranquilizer

RANGE: Native to British Columbia, and Saskatchewan to Maritimes

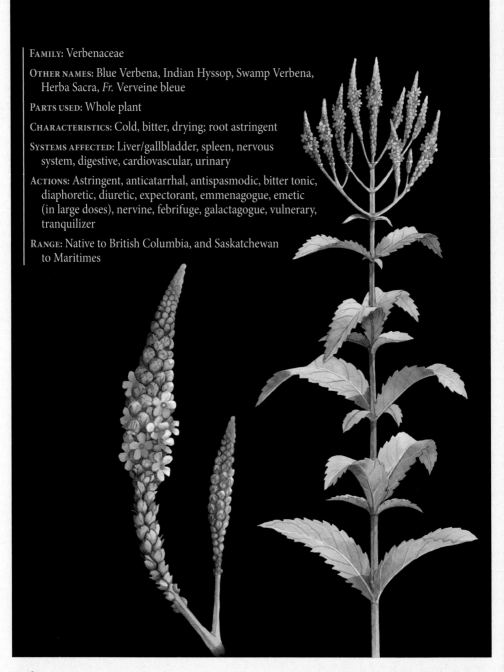

This common weed native to North America is similar in medicinal properties to the European variety *Verbena officinalis*. It is a tall, erect, branching perennial that grows from 0.6 to 1.5 metres high with intense blue-violet flower spikes and a reddish square stem and opposite lanceolate leaves that are conspicuously veined and coarsely serrated. It blooms from mid to late summer, each flower spike being up to 13 cm. long, the individual flowers having 5 lobes and no noticeable scent. It grows in ditches and along roadsides and in pastures throughout Canada, and makes a nice addition to gardens. Harvest when the plants come into bloom, tincture fresh or dry quickly in a cool, dark place for later use in teas.

MEDICINAL USES:

Colds, headaches, pain, anxiety, bleeding gums, arthritis, insomnia

- May help chest congestion, colds, fevers, chronic bronchitis, sore throats, and other respiratory infections.
- Can be a muscle relaxant and pain reliever, anti-inflammatory, can help to relieve stress headaches and swelling and inflammation from gout or arthritis.
- Helps protect the liver and kidneys, may relieve the pain from kidney stones and bladder infections.
- Used as a relaxing nervine, to reduce stress and anxiety and help with insomnia, as well as for tension in the stomach due to suppression of emotions.
- Gentle astringent for soothing inflamed and bleeding gums. Helps teething babies. Used externally for minor wounds, sores, eczema.
- Promotes milk production in nursing mothers, balances hormones, good for menstrual pain, PMS and hot flashes.

FOLKLORE: Once believed to have magical properties. Druids and sorcerers used the European variety in their rites and incantations; it was used in love charms, as it was said to have aphrodisiac qualities. Called Herba Sacra, priests used it in rituals as it was supposedly used to staunch the wounds of Jesus. It was often worn around the neck for good luck and to ward off headaches.

INFUSION: Because of its bitter taste, it's best blended with other herbs like Chamomile or Holy Basil, or for headaches with Goldenrod flowers and Mullein. For nerves, mix 4 parts Skullcap, 2 parts Motherwort, and 1 part Blue Vervain.

TINCTURE: Fresh 1:2, dry 1:4, in 40% alcohol. Take 1–2 ml., 2–4 times a day.

CAUTION: No known side effects, except slight nausea and danger of miscarriage if taken in large doses.

BOGBEAN

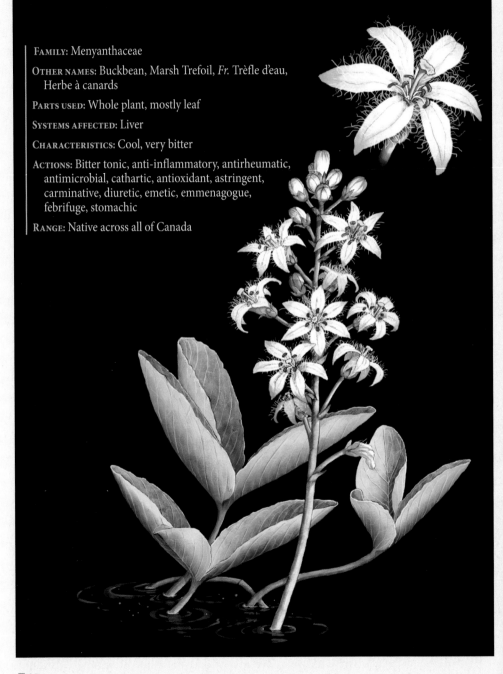

Menyanthes trifoliata

FAMILY: Menyanthaceae

OTHER NAMES: Buckbean, Marsh Trefoil, *Fr.* Trèfle d'eau, Herbe à canards

PARTS USED: Whole plant, mostly leaf

SYSTEMS AFFECTED: Liver

CHARACTERISTICS: Cool, very bitter

ACTIONS: Bitter tonic, anti-inflammatory, antirheumatic, antimicrobial, cathartic, antioxidant, astringent, carminative, diuretic, emetic, emmenagogue, febrifuge, stomachic

RANGE: Native across all of Canada

As its name suggests, this native plant grows in wetlands, ponds, bogs, swamps, and marshes. It has been used for centuries in both Europe and North America as a digestive tonic and to relieve joint pain. The stalk is usually up to 30 cm. high, rising above the water and topped with 3 smooth, oval leaflets with smooth or toothed edges. Flower stalks produce clusters of rank-smelling white or pinkish star-shaped flowers, each about 1.3 cm. wide with 5 or 6 pointed lobes covered in white hairs. They bloom from late May into June. The fruit are oval capsules containing tiny yellowish seeds that float on the water when released. Gather the leaves in early to late summer, leaving the roots intact to keep the colony healthy.

MEDICINAL USES:

Digestive and liver disorders, arthritic and rheumatic conditions, chronic infections, exhaustion and debility

- Very bitter digestive tonic, relieves digestive disturbances due to sluggishness and liver disorders, tonifies the digestive tract and increases flow of saliva and digestive juices. Relieves chronic diarrhea and stimulates bile production. Helps indigestion, hypoacidosis, bloating, and flatulence.
- May help with minor arthritic pain, gout or rheumatism, muscular pain, weakness, exhaustion, fibromyalgia and debility. Can assist with anorexia, or where there is a problem gaining weight, with lack of appetite and low vitality. Use in small doses.
- Infusion can be taken internally or used as a poultice for muscle pain and arthritis.

OTHER USES:
- Leaves were once used as a substitute for hops in beer-making.
- Powdered roots can be mixed with flour for making bread.

INFUSION: For a digestive tonic, add 1 tsp. herb to 1 cup boiling water, cover and simmer for 10 minutes. Take ½ cup 20 minutes before meals. Good for those with food sensitivities, bloating, or slow digestion.

TINCTURE: Fresh 1:2, dry 1:5, in 50% alcohol. Take 10–30 drops, 3 times a day.

COMBINATIONS:

Usually combined with other digestive herbs such as Celery seed, Gentian, Calamus, and White Willow.

CAUTION: Avoid in large doses. May irritate the digestive tract, especially if there is gastric inflammation, ulcers, diarrhea, colitis, or infection, as it stimulates production of hydrochloric acid. May cause vomiting or have a laxative effect. Avoid use if pregnant due to lack of studies.

BORAGE

Borago officinalis

FAMILY: Boraginaceae

OTHER NAMES: Starflower, Beeplant, Beebush, *Fr.* Bourrache

PARTS USED: Flowers, leaves, seeds

CHARACTERISTICS: Cooling, moistening, slightly sweet

SYSTEMS AFFECTED: Lungs, heart

ACTIONS: Aperient, diuretic, diaphoretic, demulcent, febrifuge, emollient, anti-inflammatory, expectorant, galactagogue, adrenal tonic, antidepressant

RANGE: Introduced, British Columbia to Manitoba

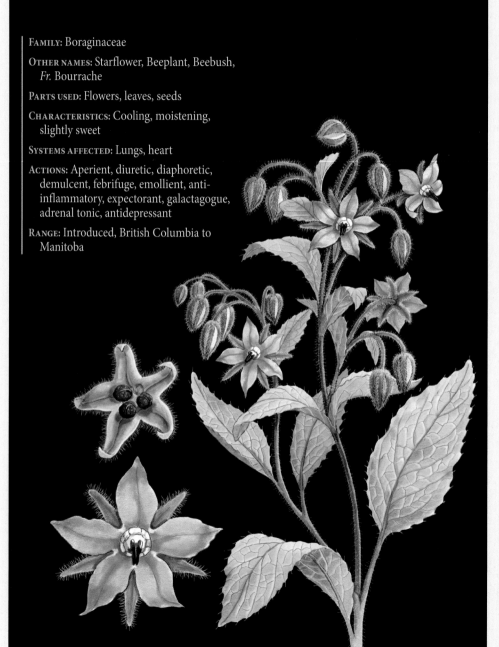

This pretty blue annual flower, traditionally served in wine before going off to battle, was once known for its ability to instill bravery and banish melancholy. Whether it was the wine or the flowers that gave soldiers courage, we can't be sure, but it continued to be used up until the last century and is still prescribed by some herbalists for depression and other ailments. It is believed to have originated in Syria and spread throughout southern Europe and north Africa, eventually becoming naturalized and cultivated by colonists in North America. A robust annual with hollow reddish or green stems and thick, wrinkled leaves, it is almost entirely covered in hairs, except for the striking blue flowers, which bloom from June to October. The plant grows from 60 to 90 cm. in height, has alternate oval leaves, and has flowers with 5 petals in the form of a star, 5 hairy sepals, and prominent black anthers, which are replaced by 3–4 brown nutlets. It is widely cultivated for its seed oil, which is rich in a fatty acid used to fight inflammation. Leaves should be picked on a sunny day before the flowers have opened and preferably used fresh, although the leaves may be dried for later use. Flowers can be picked right after blooming and may be dried, candied, or frozen into ice cubes. Keep from direct light and use within 3 months.

MEDICINAL USES:

Asthma, arthritis, skin conditions, cerebral arteriosclerosis, lung infections, urinary disorders

- Seed oil is the richest plant source of gamma-linolenic acid (GLA), an unsaturated fatty acid (omega-6) that is anti-inflammatory and boosts immunity. May lessen symptoms in people with rheumatoid arthritis, memory loss, heart conditions, menopause, gingivitis, diabetes, PMS, breast pain, asthma, and some autoimmune disorders, although there needs to be more research done to verify these claims.
- Used as a poultice or infused oil, it can help chronic inflammatory skin diseases like eczema, dermatitis, and psoriasis, reduces itch, and treats insect bites, rashes, sores, ringworm.
- Natural sedative, adrenal tonic, causes a significant reduction in anxiety and restores balance to the nervous system. Specific for neurasthenia, added to formulas for depression. Can help with hyperthyroidism, and to reduce stress and tension.
- Reduces inflammation of arthritis, lessens swelling and pain.
- Increases effectiveness of other medications used for urinary and respiratory disorders, arthritis, and skin diseases.

OTHER USES:
- Flowers are added to salads, drinks or confections; young leaves have a cucumber-like flavour, may also be used in salads or teas.
- Beneficial for gardens as it is rich in nitrogen and other plant nutrients; it attracts bees and also aphids, which can keep them off other plants.

TINCTURE: Standard, use dried leaves and flowers. Take 6–15 drops 3 times a day.

CAUTION: Plant contains pyrrolizidine alkaloids, which can be toxic to the liver and aggravate cirrhosis, hepatitis, and other liver ailments. Only use seed oil that is labelled as non-hepatotoxic or PA free. Avoid if pregnant or lactating. Not for children under 12. Avoid long-term use, large doses. Contact with leaves may cause dermatitis in a small number of people.

BURDOCK

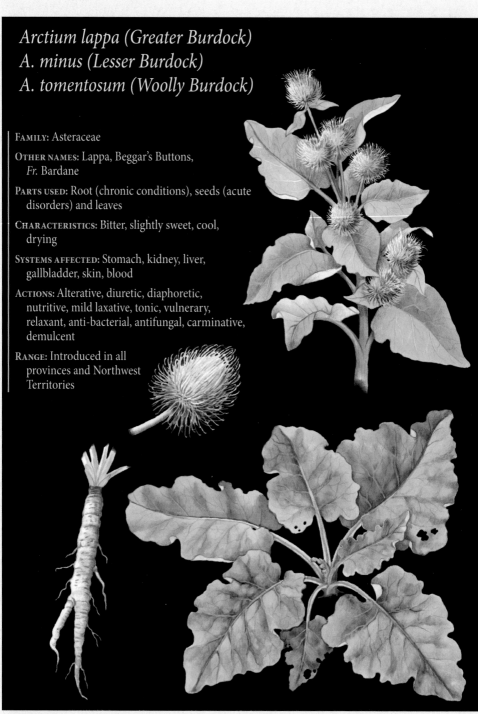

Arctium lappa (Greater Burdock)
A. minus (Lesser Burdock)
A. tomentosum (Woolly Burdock)

FAMILY: Asteraceae

OTHER NAMES: Lappa, Beggar's Buttons, *Fr.* Bardane

PARTS USED: Root (chronic conditions), seeds (acute disorders) and leaves

CHARACTERISTICS: Bitter, slightly sweet, cool, drying

SYSTEMS AFFECTED: Stomach, kidney, liver, gallbladder, skin, blood

ACTIONS: Alterative, diuretic, diaphoretic, nutritive, mild laxative, tonic, vulnerary, relaxant, anti-bacterial, antifungal, carminative, demulcent

RANGE: Introduced in all provinces and Northwest Territories

Burdock is another one of those pesky weeds people hate having on their property, mainly because of its burrs, which will attach to just about anything, particularly house pets. However, it's one of the best detoxifying herbs. It grows mainly in waste places, meadows, and woods and can grow up to 1.8 metres tall. The lower leaves are large, wavy, and heart-shaped, covered with fine hairs, and light grey on the underside. The upper leaves are smaller and oval-shaped with less of the downy covering. The flowerheads are purple and enclosed in a round spiny shell with prickles that hook onto everything that passes by. The long taproot is collected after the first year of growth in early spring, sliced and dried quickly for later use, or eaten fresh as a vegetable. For the best texture, harvest the roots that grow in soft, loamy soil. Do not confuse with Rhubarb leaves, which are toxic.

MEDICINAL USES:

Skin diseases, blood purification, urinary problems, arthritis, PMS

- Contains many minerals, especially iron, that make it valuable for the blood. Beneficial as a detoxifier and blood and liver tonic, as it promotes sweating and detoxifies the epidermal tissues, assists in absorption of nutrients, aids digestion, and relieves bloating and water retention. It works best if used in moderate doses over a long period of time. The seed is said to be better used for acute illnesses, whereas the root is more beneficial for chronic problems of the kidneys, bladder, skin, and bowel, and is more permanent.
- Alleviates the pain of arthritis, rheumatism, sciatica, and lumbago by its diuretic action, which increases the removal of urine and toxic substances.
- Due to its ability to increase circulation to the skin and its mucilaginous, demulcent nature, it helps chronic skin eruptions like acne, psoriasis, eczema, boils, and herpes. It can be taken internally in an infusion and/or used externally as a wash or poultice. Crushed seed can be poulticed on bruises, and the leaves can be used on burns, ulcers, or sores, on the forehead to relieve headache, or on the scalp to relieve itchiness or dandruff. Studies have shown it may even inhibit cancer growth.
- Digestive herb, the bitterness in the leaf can stimulate bile production, cleanse the liver, and repair the damaging effects of alcohol. The demulcent quality soothes the digestive tract and contains inulin, which feeds healthy bacteria.
- Eliminates harmful acids from the kidneys, improves filtration, and may heal cystitis.
- Regulates the menstrual cycle, relieves mastitis and menopausal symptoms, eases swollen prostate glands.

OTHER USES:
- The stalk, when cut before the flower opens, peeled, and boiled, makes a tasty vegetable.
- The young leaves can be eaten in salads, but are slightly laxative.
- The root may be boiled and eaten like carrots. It can also be fermented and made into kimchi with grated ginger and carrots.

DECOCTION: 2 tsp. dried root in 2 cups boiling water, soak overnight, boil again and simmer 5–10 minutes. Drink 3 times a day.

TINCTURE: Fresh root 1:2, dried 1:5, in 60% alcohol. Take 30–90 drops 3 times a day.

COMBINATIONS:

Burdock and Red Clover make a good blood tonic. Burdock can be combined with Yellow Dock or Dandelion root to detoxify and stimulate digestion.

CAUTION: When gathering seeds, be careful to remove the splinters clinging to them before use as they can be extremely irritant.

CALENDULA

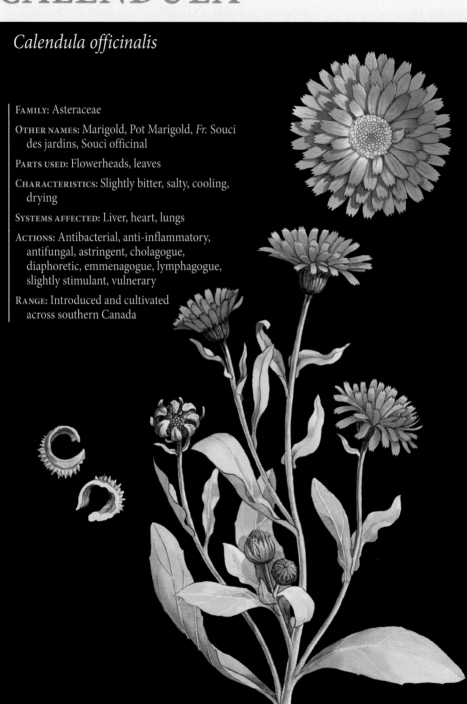

Calendula officinalis

FAMILY: Asteraceae

OTHER NAMES: Marigold, Pot Marigold, *Fr.* Souci des jardins, Souci officinal

PARTS USED: Flowerheads, leaves

CHARACTERISTICS: Slightly bitter, salty, cooling, drying

SYSTEMS AFFECTED: Liver, heart, lungs

ACTIONS: Antibacterial, anti-inflammatory, antifungal, astringent, cholagogue, diaphoretic, emmenagogue, lymphagogue, slightly stimulant, vulnerary

RANGE: Introduced and cultivated across southern Canada

This common annual garden herb is a native of Southern Europe and Asia which was brought to America by settlers for its pretty blooms and valuable medicinal qualities. It has a branching, slightly hairy stem about 30 cm. high, with alternate lance-shaped leaves and a large solitary terminal flowerhead on each stem. The 3-toothed petals are actually ray florets, or individual flowers grouped together, and range in colour from bright yellow and orange to russet red. Do not confuse Calendula with Garden Marigolds of the genus *Tagetes*, which are often planted in gardens to repel pests due to their unpleasant smell.

Pick the entire flowerhead for medicines, as many of the medicinal constituents are found in the green bases or calyxes; however, only the petals should be used if eating them raw in salads, as the small hairs on the calyx can be irritating. They should be picked often to encourage new growth, and only after the dew has evaporated, then dried on screens out of the sun for 7–10 days.

MEDICINAL USES:

Skin problems, wounds, varicose veins, digestive problems, swollen lymph nodes, periodontal disease

- Compresses soaked in diluted tincture or infusion help heal abscesses, scalds, ulcers, cracked nipples, stings, sprains, diaper rash, and minor wounds. It helps prevent infection, gangrene, and pus formation, relieves swelling and redness, and speeds healing.
- Useful for healing varicose veins, both as a compress and internally to relieve swelling, pain, and inflammation.
- Effective internally for digestive issues such as GERD, peptic ulcers, Crohn's, colitis, and gastritis; relieves pain and heals mucous tissue in the digestive tract.
- Stimulates the lymphatic system; reduces acute or chronic swelling of the lymph nodes from infections, helps build immunity.
- Used in a mouthwash for thrush, bleeding gums, periodontal disease.
- Crushed calyx and flower stems can be applied to skin and covered with a bandage to help dissolve warts and corns.
- Brings on suppressed menstruation.

OTHER USES:
- A rinse adds golden highlights to hair.
- Boiled flowers create a yellow dye for fabrics.
- Cheap alternative for saffron in cooking.

TINCTURE: Fresh plant 1:2 or dried 1:5, with 70% alcohol. Take 5–30 drops 3 times a day. Dilute with at least 3 parts water for topical use.

INFUSION: 1 tbsp. dry herb in 1 cup boiling water, take 3 times a day.

SALVE: Combine macerated oils of Calendula, Plantain, Chickweed, St. John's Wort, and Violet; heat gently, adding just enough beeswax to solidify the oils (usually 28 grams beeswax to 1 cup oil). When melted, remove from heat and add several drops of Vitamin E and essential oil if desired. Pour into jars.

CAUTION: Not for use during pregnancy. May cause allergic reaction in sensitive individuals. Do not eat raw flower base (calyx) as it could be irritant to mouth and digestive tract.

CASCARA SAGRADA

Frangula purshiana

FAMILY: Rhamnaceae

OTHER NAMES: Cascara Buckthorn, Chittam Bark, Sacred Bark, *Fr.* Nerprun cascara

PARTS USED: Aged bark

CHARACTERISTICS: Bitter, cooling

SYSTEMS AFFECTED: Stomach, liver, gallbladder, spleen, intestines

ACTIONS: Laxative, tonic, alterative, hepatic, stimulant, nervine

RANGE: Native to southern British Columbia

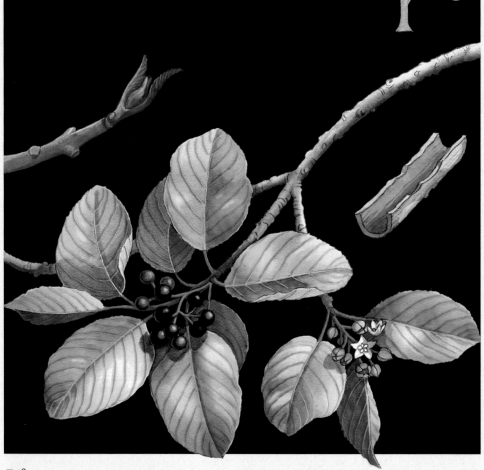

This deciduous shrub, the largest belonging to the Buckthorn family, has been used as a laxative for hundreds of years by natives and Spanish settlers, who gave it the name Cascara Sagrada, Spanish for "sacred bark," because of its use as medicine. It usually grows only 5–10 metres tall; however, it has been known to reach 15 metres. Its outer bark is light grey or brown and often spotted with lichens, the inner bark an orange-yellow, and it is usually found in wet, shady places, along streams or coastlines. In winter it grows small, hairy, rusty-brown buds resembling two angel wings, which in spring grow into shiny green, oval, alternate leaves which are sparsely serrated. The inconspicuous white flowers emerge in May or June, followed by green berries that turn red and eventually black. The best time to harvest is late spring to early summer. This shrub is endangered, so do not strip the bark from the trunk; instead, remove a branch of about one centimetre thick and strip the bark off as soon as possible. Use gloves, as the inner bark is extremely potent and can penetrate the skin. It should be left to dry in a paper bag for at least 1 year or up to 3 years before using, as it is too strong to consume fresh and will cause cramping, nausea, and diarrhea.

MEDICINAL USES:

Constipation, lack of appetite, digestive sluggishness, toxic liver, leaky gut

- Contains anthraquinone glycosides, which stimulate contractions in the intestinal wall, increasing peristalsis and strengthening the lower intestine to relieve acute or chronic constipation. Take before bed; it usually requires 8 hours to work.
- Smaller doses will tonify the colon and should be taken in combination with carminatives like fresh Ginger to reduce cramping, and/or Aniseed, Fennel, or Cardamom to ease nausea and mask the intense bitterness. People with chronic constipation need to modify their diet and eliminate processed and refined foods.
- Smaller doses taken 10–15 minutes before meals stimulate digestion and increase appetite, releasing enzymes from the pancreas, liver, and duodenum. Can prevent acid reflux, help detoxify the liver, and aid in repairing the intestinal wall where there is leaky gut syndrome. May relieve hemorrhoids caused by constipation and straining. Some herbalists claim that it will release stuck emotional issues as well.
- Unlike other products, Cascara Sagrada taken daily in small doses will not create a dependency, and is one of the safest laxatives. However, you should drink plenty of water while taking it.

OTHER USES:
- This hardwood is dense and strong, making it ideal for tool handles.
- After being dried and seasoned, the wood also makes excellent charcoal for cooking.

TINCTURE: Take 1 tsp. before bed as a laxative. To use as a bitter digestive tonic, take 1–5 drops 10–15 minutes before meals. Combine with fresh Ginger, Aniseed, Licorice root, Fennel and/or Cardamom.

CAUTION: Not for use during pregnancy. Fresh bark will cause intense cramping, diarrhea and/or vomiting. Dry for 1–3 years before using. Long-term use may result in loss of electrolytes, especially potassium, and dependency. Avoid with inflammatory bowel disorders or obstructions.

CATNIP

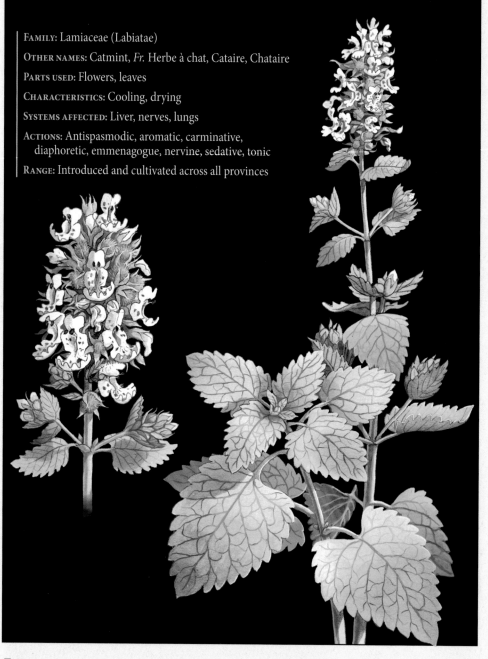

Nepeta cataria

Family: Lamiaceae (Labiatae)

Other names: Catmint, *Fr.* Herbe à chat, Cataire, Chataire

Parts used: Flowers, leaves

Characteristics: Cooling, drying

Systems affected: Liver, nerves, lungs

Actions: Antispasmodic, aromatic, carminative, diaphoretic, emmenagogue, nervine, sedative, tonic

Range: Introduced and cultivated across all provinces

Everyone knows about the ability of this herb to drive cats crazy. I tried to grow Catnip for years, but all I succeeded in doing was attracting all the felines in the neighbourhood to come over and roll in my garden in a drunken frenzy. I have stopped trying, although they say it's better to plant seeds; apparently as long as the plants aren't bruised, the essential oils that attract cats are not released, but I'm not convinced. Short of installing an iron cage around each plant and deep in the ground, I suspect the cats will get at them one way or another.

Most people have no idea this hardy perennial is also a medicinal plant, brought to America from Europe, Africa, and Asia as a garden plant. It has since escaped to the wild, and is found near roadsides, fields, and streams, but is easy to grow from seed if you can keep the cats away from it. It resembles mint, belonging to the same family, only Catnip has more of a citrusy aroma. Leaves are opposite, toothed and heart-shaped, and the flowers, which grow from July often into October, are white, light blue, or purple, often with pink spots, and tubular. Harvest the flowering tops when in full bloom and dry for later use.

MEDICINAL USES:

Cold and flu, upset stomach, colic, cramps, nervousness and stress, amenorrhea and dysmenorrhea, toothache, skin irritation

- A relaxing, mild, aromatic herb that settles the stomach, calms nerves, and relieves gas pains, headache, motion sickness, vomiting, and trouble settling down to sleep. May be combined with Chamomile, Fennel, Lemon Balm, Spearmint, or Elderflower.
- Diaphoretic, it promotes sweating, and can relieve colds, chills, fevers, congestion, and sore throat when ingested hot in infusion. When taken in cold infusion, it becomes tonic. The Ojibwa steep it with an equal amount of Tansy for fever.
- Antispasmodic, it relieves muscle pain, menstrual cramps, and gastrointestinal cramps or IBS. It is preferable to use fresh leaf tincture.
- Used by Indigenous Peoples in preparations, particularly for children, for colds, coughs, colic, stomach upsets, diarrhea, sore throat, fever, or bronchitis.
- Mildly anesthetic, the leaf chewed or rubbed on the gums relieves toothache pain and sore gums.
- Used in a poultice for sore nipples, bruises, hives, swellings, and boils, it is a mild antibiotic and antifungal.

OTHER USES:
- Makes an effective mosquito repellant. Crush leaves and soak in vodka. Strain and put into a spray bottle.
- Young leaves are edible and can be added to salads.

TINCTURE: Fresh leaves 1:2, dried 1:5, in 50% alcohol. Take ¼–1 tsp. up to 4 times a day.

INFUSION: 1 heaped teaspoon in 1 cup water steeped for 10 minutes, up to 4 times a day.

GASTRITIS INFUSION: Combine 2 parts Catnip, 2 parts Fennel seed, and 1 part Licorice root. Use 1–2 tsp. in 1 cup boiling water, infuse covered for 10–15 minutes.

CAUTION: Not for use during pregnancy. Very large doses may induce vomiting and dizziness.

CELANDINE

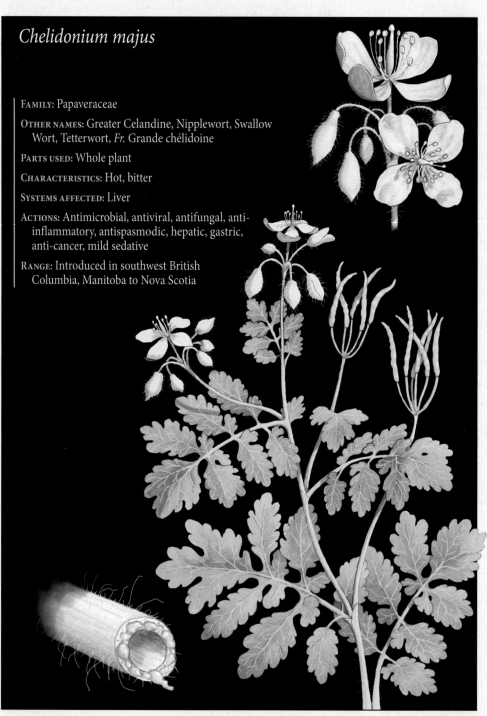

Chelidonium majus

Family: Papaveraceae

Other names: Greater Celandine, Nipplewort, Swallow Wort, Tetterwort, *Fr.* Grande chélidoine

Parts used: Whole plant

Characteristics: Hot, bitter

Systems affected: Liver

Actions: Antimicrobial, antiviral, antifungal, anti-inflammatory, antispasmodic, hepatic, gastric, anti-cancer, mild sedative

Range: Introduced in southwest British Columbia, Manitoba to Nova Scotia

This biennial is originally a native of Europe, Asia, and North Africa and has a long history as a herbal medicine both there and in North America. Its name derives from the Greek word *chelidon*, meaning "swallow," a bird that, according to folklore, arrived every year just as the flower began to bloom and fed it to their nestlings to improve their sight. It is very similar to our native Celandine Poppy (*Stylophorum diphyllum*), which has larger and showier flowers but no known medicinal use. Celandine grows at the edge of forests, in lowlands, foothills, and along roadsides, often reaching a metre in height. Its leaves are compound, alternate, lobed, and toothed, with a cluster of 2 to 6 bright yellow 4-petalled flowers at the end of a branched, sparsely hairy stem. When broken, the stems exude a yellow-orange latex sap rich in alkaloids and proteins that can be irritating to some people. The above-ground parts can be picked during the flowering season and used fresh or dried quickly in an oven. Roots may be dug in the fall and used fresh or recently dried.

MEDICINAL USES:
Liver congestion, indigestion, gallbladder complaints, toothache, eye inflammation, warts, corns

- Used for centuries in Europe for liver sluggishness, indigestion, gallbladder inflammation and stones, hepatitis, and jaundice, characterized by pain and tenderness in the upper abdomen, dull pain beneath the right shoulder blade, and a yellow tinge to the skin. It thins the bile and increases secretion, as well as reducing intestinal spasms, making it easier to expel stones and prevent their formation. However, recent testing has concluded that caution is necessary due to possible liver toxicity with this herb. It should only be used under supervision by a professional and in the proper doses. It is considered safe for short-term use to treat flatulence and dyspepsia. A careful diet is necessary when taking any liver-cleansing herb; avoid junk food, alcohol, excess sugar, and unhealthy fats.
- Typically the juice and yellow latex were used in folk medicine for eye inflammation, getting rid of warts, corns and calluses, eczema, boils, and rashes. The root was often chewed to relieve toothache.
- Anecdotal evidence suggests that taking a decoction of Celandine for 2 weeks may cause significant reduction of cancer tissue in squamous cell carcinoma of the esophagus, and possibly stomach cancer, but more research needs to be done.
- May be effective used as an antispasmodic in a syrup in cases of chronic bronchitis and whooping cough.

TINCTURE: Fresh plant 1:2 with 50% alcohol, 10–25 drops a day.

INFUSION: ½ to 1 tsp. powdered root or herb in 1 cup boiling water, infuse 30 minutes. Drink cool, ½ cup per day.

JUICE: For warts or corns, dab with fresh juice 2 or 3 times a day.

COMBINATIONS:

Barberry, Dandelion root, and Burdock for liver congestion

CAUTION: Not for use during pregnancy or lactation. May cause liver toxicity, especially if taking other pharmaceuticals or liver medications; discontinue use if symptoms worsen. Sap can be irritant, use gloves when handling. Can stimulate an immune response so may decrease effectiveness of immunosuppressants. Not recommended for very young children or the elderly. Use only under supervision of a healthcare professional and for a short term only.

CHICKWEED

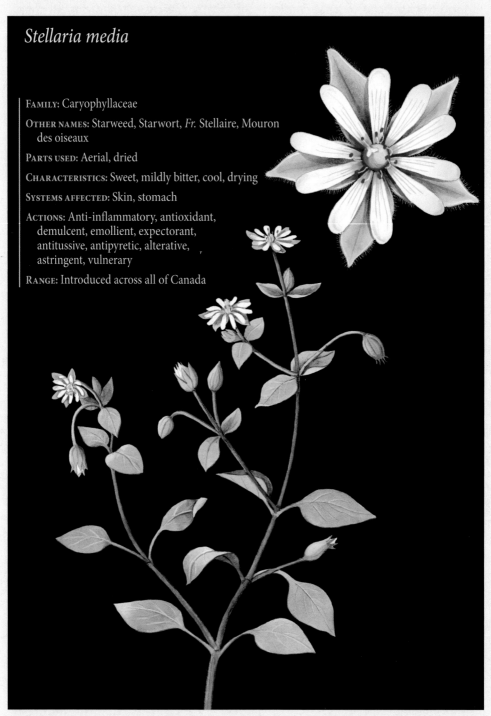

Stellaria media

Family: Caryophyllaceae

Other names: Starweed, Starwort, *Fr.* Stellaire, Mouron des oiseaux

Parts used: Aerial, dried

Characteristics: Sweet, mildly bitter, cool, drying

Systems affected: Skin, stomach

Actions: Anti-inflammatory, antioxidant, demulcent, emollient, expectorant, antitussive, antipyretic, alterative, astringent, vulnerary

Range: Introduced across all of Canada

Chickweed is a small, creeping plant, growing up to 30 cm. high with weak, many-branched stems that trail along the ground. Its name, *Stellaria media*, means "little stars," which perfectly describes its flowers. It is identified by a line of hairs running up one side of the stem then continuing along the opposite side when it reaches a pair of leaves. The opposite leaves are succulent, smooth, oval, and pointed. The small white flowers have 5 petals that are deeply divided, seeming like there are 10 petals, and are only open for 12 hours, on fine days. In the rain they droop, and at night the leaves fold over the delicate flowers and protect the tip of the shoot. They begin blooming in early spring and continue through till the fall. The seedpod is a small capsule with teeth that, once ripe, shake the seeds when the wind blows. It grows in fields and waste areas and should be collected between May and July. It is often mistaken for Grass-leaved Stitchwort (*Stellaria graminea*), which is hairless and has grass-shaped leaves, and Mouse-eared Chickweed (*Cerastium ssp.*), which has densely hairy leaves. Neither has the same medicinal properties as *Stellaria media*.

MEDICINAL USES:

Skin irritations, weight loss, sore throat, respiratory infections, fever, inflammation

- Whole plant is edible, nutritious, high in vitamins and minerals, may be added to a salad or used as a potherb. Contains saponins, which improve absorption of nutrients. Works well as a cleansing herb and spring tonic. Helps in weight loss, is mildly diuretic and laxative.
- In the form of an ointment or poultice it has a cooling and drying effect on skin irritations, itches, rashes, wounds, ulcers, boils, eczema, and psoriasis. A fresh poultice will actually heat up as it draws out infection from the body. Its emollient properties make it very soothing. As a decoction it can be used to treat rheumatic pain, wounds, or ulcers. It may also be added to bathwater to soothe inflammation, sunburn, or hemorrhoids. Tincture of the fresh herb has been used successfully to dissolve cysts and benign tumors.
- Treats fevers, inflammation, and other hot diseases. Soothes sore throat and reduces swelling and irritation in the sinuses as well as easing respiratory tract and reproductive inflammations.

POULTICE: Apply fresh chopped herb directly onto sores or wounds, cover with a clean towel, and leave for up to 3 hours. Replace if poultice begins to feel warm. If using older plants, cook in water and cool before applying.

INFUSION: Mix 4 tbsp. of fresh herb with 2½ cups boiling water, infuse 10 minutes, strain. Drink throughout the day. Great for people recovering from an illness.

TINCTURE: Fill a jar with fresh chopped herb, cover with vodka, and let it sit for at least 6 weeks. Use one dropperful 2 or 3 times a day for several months.

OIL: Macerate fresh or dried herb in olive oil for 4 days, then squeeze through cheesecloth. Combines well with Yarrow or St. John's Wort oils.

CHOKECHERRY

Prunus virginiana

FAMILY: Rosaceae

OTHER NAMES: Black Chokecherry, Bitterberry, *Fr.* Cerisier de Virginie

PARTS USED: Bark, berries, inner bark, and roots

CHARACTERISTICS: Cooling

SYSTEMS AFFECTED: Lungs, stomach, circulatory

ACTIONS: Astringent, blood tonic, sedative, appetite stimulant, pectoral

RANGE: Native across all provinces

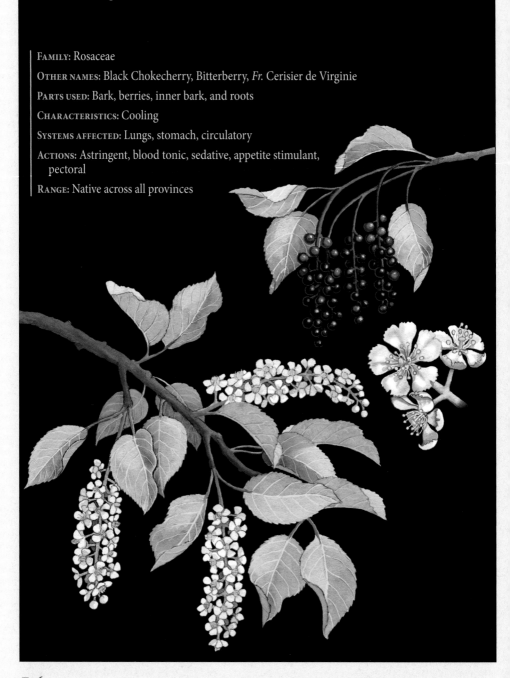

As you might expect, Chokecherry gets its name from its bitter, sour taste, which will make your mouth pucker from its astringency, particularly when eaten raw. But despite its reputation, it has been used by Indigenous Peoples for hundreds of years, both as a food and a medicine. It grows as a shrub or small tree, usually 6 to 9 metres tall, has oval, finely toothed leaves, and is easily identified by its flowers, which grow in racemes of up to 10 cm. long late in the spring. The red berries hang in drupes, turning to black as they mature. Each berry contains a single seed, which is considered toxic not only to humans but particularly to livestock, which may eat them and the leaves in large quantities, often causing sickness and death. Avoid confusing Chokecherry with Chokeberry from the *Aronia* genus; the latter grows in short bunches, a berry contains several seeds, and its leaves are more oblong. Bark and berries of the Chokecherry should be dried before using.

MEDICINAL USES:

Respiratory tract infections, fever, childbirth, stomach upset, diarrhea, skin sores

- Seeds, leaves and bark contain amygdalin, which hydrolyzes into hydrocyanic acid, which in small quantities can stimulate respiration and improve digestion, however in excess it can cause respiratory failure and even death. Its healing and nutritive properties are well known by Indigenous people, who add the dried berries to their pemmican, consisting of dried meat (usually bison), bone marrow, and lard ground together, dried into cakes, and stored over the winter. Boiling or drying the berries or bark neutralizes the toxins.
- Some Indigenous Peoples also use the bark and berries during childbirth as a sedative to relieve labour pains and ease anxiety, and the astringency reduces the chance of hemorrhaging.
- Used as a digestive tonic, the bark and berries increase appetite and tone the circulation during convalescence, and relieve dyspepsia, ulcers, bleeding in the bowel, and diarrhea. The seeds have been found to contain some anti-cancer properties, although very little research has been done. Often combined with other digestive herbs such as Licorice, Ginseng, and Anise in tinctures to relieve digestive weakness.
- Excellent remedy for irritating spasmodic coughs and colds, bronchitis, persistent fevers, sore throat, and headache. Often the berries are used to make cough syrup.
- Powder or infusion of the black bark can be used for burns, sores, and ulcers.

OTHER USES:
- Green dye made from leaves and inner bark, purple dye from the fruit.
- Berries used to make jams, jellies, pies, syrup, and wine.
- Wood used in construction, to make arrows, or for carving pipe stems.

TINCTURE: Bark 1:5 with 60% alcohol, 30–90 drops up to 3 times a day.

INFUSION: Standard infusion or decoction, ¼–½ cups up to 3 times a day.

CHOKECHERRY JELLY: Put about 8 cups cleaned Chokecherries with 1½ cups water in a pot. Boil and simmer until berries are soft and mushy. Mash, cool, and pour through a sieve or cheesecloth, squeezing as much as possible. Add 1 cup sugar for every cup of juice (about 4 cups) plus 1 tbsp. lemon juice. Boil about 30 minutes or until it reaches gel stage. Pour into sterilized jars.

CAUTION: Seeds, bark, and leaves contain amygdalin, which breaks down into hydrocyanic acid, a toxin to humans and livestock. Boil before using, and add sugar to lessen toxicity. Use with caution.

CLUBMOSS

Lycopodium clavatum

FAMILY: Lycopodiaceae

OTHER NAMES: Staghorn, Running Clubmoss, Ground Pine, Wolf's Claw, Foxtail, *Fr.* Lycopode claviforme, Courants verts

PARTS USED: Spores

SYSTEMS AFFECTED: Urinary, digestive

ACTIONS: Analgesic, antioxidant, anti-inflammatory, antimicrobial, diuretic, nervine, neuroprotective, stomachic

RANGE: Native across Canada, except Alberta and Northwest Territories

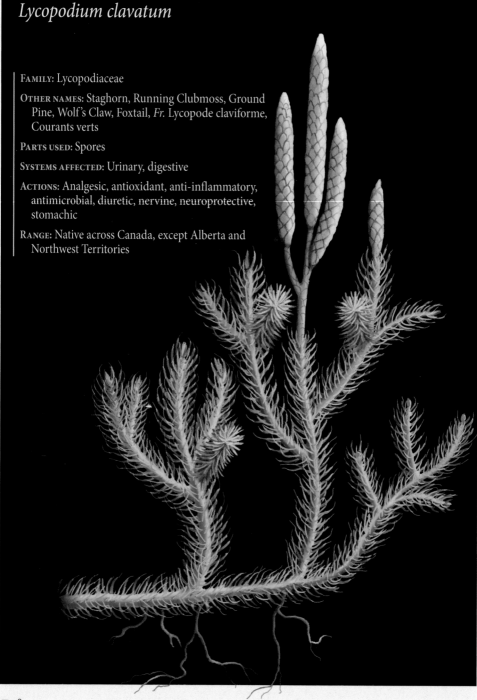

Clubmoss is a creeping evergreen found all over the world, related to primitive plants that flourished millions of years ago. Unrelated to true mosses, it grows close to the ground in woods, fields, and tundra, sending up vertical branches that look like pine seedlings. Although the entire plant was once used, it's mostly just the spores that have been used since the seventeenth century, as the plant contains toxins that can be harmful. The tops are carefully removed late in the summer and then shaken to release the fine powder, which should then be sifted to remove extraneous matter.

MEDICINAL USES:

Edema, constipation, diarrhea, gout, rheumatism, urinary and kidney disorders, gastric inflammation, and indigestion

- For many years the spores were used primarily as a dusting powder for skin diseases like eczema, herpes, and ulcers. It can prevent chafing in infants and relieve irritation, stop nosebleeds, and aid in wound healing.
- Used as a diuretic in cases of edema, helps cases of gout, rheumatism, and arthritis, relieves bladder and kidney irritation, cystitis, and blood in the urine.
- Helps digestive issues, controlling both diarrhea and constipation, stomach inflammation, liver complaints, and indigestion.
- Recent studies have shown the Lycopodium genus contains huperzine A, a compound that may be useful in treating memory loss, Alzheimer's, and dementia; however, particularly with *Lycopodium serratum*, commonly used in Chinese medicine, there are risks of toxicity to the liver. Much more research is needed.

OTHER USES:
- Powder forms a water-repellant barrier useful in treating some skin diseases where the skin needs to remain dry, and to coat pills to keep them from sticking together.
- The spores will explode when ignited and was once used as flash powder in early photography or for magic tricks.

COMFREY

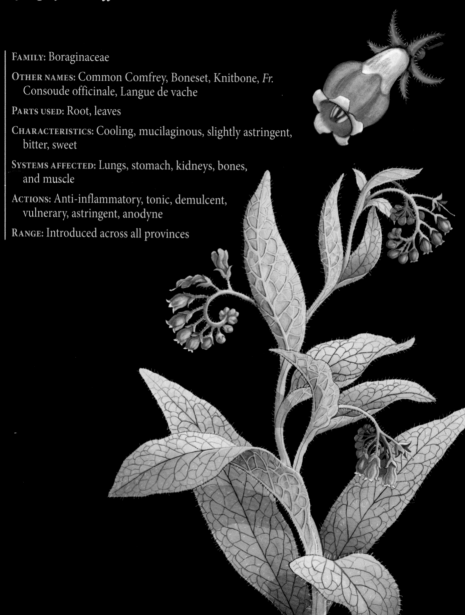

Symphytum officinale

FAMILY: Boraginaceae

OTHER NAMES: Common Comfrey, Boneset, Knitbone, *Fr.* Consoude officinale, Langue de vache

PARTS USED: Root, leaves

CHARACTERISTICS: Cooling, mucilaginous, slightly astringent, bitter, sweet

SYSTEMS AFFECTED: Lungs, stomach, kidneys, bones, and muscle

ACTIONS: Anti-inflammatory, tonic, demulcent, vulnerary, astringent, anodyne

RANGE: Introduced across all provinces

This tenacious perennial, a member of the Borage family, is found across North America on moist grasslands, waste places, and old fields. Originally from Europe, it grows to a height of 30 to 90 cm. and spreads rapidly from even a small piece of the root, quickly taking over a garden. The stems and large alternate lance-shaped leaves are covered in coarse, bristly hairs, and produce a mucilaginous gel when broken. The bell-shaped flowers emerge in May and June and can vary widely in colour, from pink or purple to blue, white, and even yellow. The plant has a long history of use, both internally and externally; however, there has been much controversy among herbalists in the last few years as to whether it should be used internally due to the presence of pyrrolizidine alkaloids, which may damage the liver. Whatever your viewpoint, its use is highly valued and safe as an external medicine. The leaves are generally harvested during flowering and dried in bundles upside down out of the sun for later use. The roots may be dug up in the fall or early spring, cleaned, and cut into thin slices before drying.

MEDICINAL USES:

Broken bones, bruises, sprains, varicose veins, arthritis, sore muscles, skin ulcers

- The plant contains allantoin, a cell proliferant that speeds up the healing process and encourages new cell growth. Also contains rosmarinic acid, which is an anti-inflammatory. Particularly useful in external treatment of cuts, bruises, sores, ulcers, eczema, and other skin conditions. Preparations include salves, ointments, oils, poultices, and compresses.
- Helpful for osteoarthritis, swelling, and stiffness in the joints, acute myalgia, back pain, sprains, contusions, sports injuries. Clinical studies have proven its effectiveness; after 12 days of external treatment twice a day, most patients show a marked improvement. Fresh abrasions healed 3 days faster and myalgia pain and sprained ankles improved significantly. Wounds should be cleaned and disinfected meticulously before using as it will seal it quickly, and could cause infection or debris to be trapped in the wound. Do not use where there is pus or infection already in the wound.
- Indicated to be effective in healing bone fractures and injured tendons or ligaments more rapidly. However, bones need to be set properly before using Comfrey.
- The astringency of the root has been used internally throughout history in the form of decoctions or tinctures to stop hemorrhages and diarrhea, or as a demulcent to soothe coughs and lung problems. However, due to possible liver toxicity, it is not recommended.

OTHER USES: Leaves make an excellent compost, as they add many nutrients to the soil.

DECOCTION: Standard decoction of root used in compresses. Fresh leaves or crushed root may be applied to skin in the form of a poultice.

OIL: Macerate root and/or dried leaves in oil for 4 to 6 weeks. Filter out plant material and store out of sunlight.

COMBINATIONS:

Calendula and Plantain to help healing, Marshmallow for dry, cracked skin.

CAUTION: Contains pyrrolizidine alkaloids that may damage the liver and cause hepatic veno-occlusive disease, which creates obstructions in the veins surrounding the liver and could be life-threatening. Avoid internal use. Considered safe for use externally, but avoid using for more than 10 days at a time without guidance from a healthcare professional.

CRAMP BARK

Viburnum opulus (Cramp Bark)
Viburnum edule (Highbush Cranberry)

FAMILY: Adoxaceae (Caprifoliaceae)

OTHER NAMES: *V. opulus*: European Highbush Cranberry, Guelder Rose, American Bush Cranberry, *Fr.* Viorne obier; *V. edule*: Squashberry, Mooseberry, *Fr.* Viorne comestible

PARTS USED: Bark, root bark, berries

CHARACTERISTICS: Bitter, cool, dry, slightly acrid

SYSTEMS AFFECTED: Liver, lungs, heart, small intestine, reproductive, urinary

ACTIONS: Anti-inflammatory, anti-abortive, antispasmodic, astringent, sedative, nervine

RANGE: *V. opulus* introduced across all provinces; *V. edule* native across all of Canada

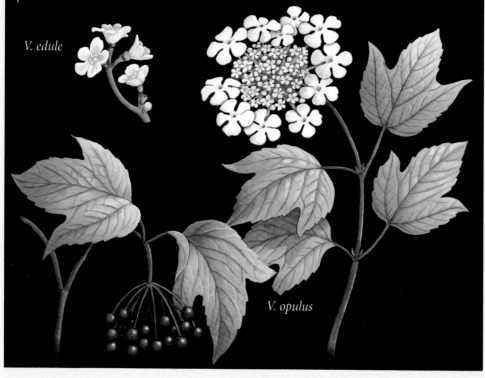

V. edule

V. opulus
var. americanum

V. opulus

V. edule

V. opulus

The name of this deciduous shrub gives an indication of its usefulness as an antispasmodic in relieving cramps and muscle pains, but its history includes many other uses. It was originally native to Europe but eventually became naturalized, and now both the European and the American variant are found in abundance across Canada, along with its native cousin *V. edule*, which has similar properties but is not as strong medicinally. Cramp Bark grows up to 4 metres in height; the 3-lobed leaves are opposite and usually serrated with a rounded base. Flower clusters are comprised of an outer ring of larger white 5-petalled sterile flowers surrounding the centre of small fertile yellowish flowers, which eventually ripen into bright red drupes of bitter-tasting berries, which tend to smell like old socks, but when cooked into jellies with oranges or apples can be quite tasty. They are incidentally not related to the true cranberry, of the Vaccinium family. The *V. edule* variety has only one type of flower, and its berries do not hang in drupes. The best way to distinguish the varieties is by the glands at the base of the leaf. The bark is the part most commonly used for medicine, peeled from the root or branches. It should be collected in spring and summer, when its properties are the strongest, and dried for later use.

MEDICINAL USES:

Cramps, muscle spasms, menstrual cramps, irritable bowel, headaches, arthritis, high blood pressure

- Antispasmodic, it helps relieve all kinds of cramps and muscle spasms and the pain associated with them. Also contains methyl salicylate, a precursor to salicylic acid, which is used in aspirin to relieve pain, but methyl salicylate is milder and can usually be used without irritation to the stomach. Relieves migraines and tension headaches.
- A uterine tonic, it eases bloating, relaxes menstrual cramps, and tones the uterine muscles. In pregnancy it can stop uterine contractions that come too early, preventing miscarriage, improving muscle tone, and strengthening the uterus for labour. It also helps return the uterus to normal after the birth and helps prevent prolapse in later years. Can be combined with Wild Yam and False Unicorn Root for an effective uterine tonic. Works best if taken 1–2 days before menstruation.
- As a fomentation, liniment, or internally as a tincture, it relieves muscle spasms, backache, chronic muscle tension, and restless legs.
- Has a cardiotonic effect, toning blood vessels, causing the heart to beat stronger, and lowering blood pressure and heart rate. Eases heart palpitations. Relaxes without being sedating.
- Relieves asthma and spasmodic coughing, and astringency dries mucosal tissue.
- Eases discomfort from urinary tract infections, IBS, diarrhea, indigestion.

OTHER USES:
- Berries are rich in vitamins C and K and can be used in jellies, syrups, and jams.
- A red dye can be made from the fruit.

DECOCTION: 2 tbsp. per cup of water; Ginger or other spices may be added to mask the taste. Take 6–8 tbsp. 4 times a day, or use in a fomentation or compress.

TINCTURE: Bark 1:5 with 50% alcohol, 20–50 drops 4 times a day or as needed.

CAUTION: Avoid with low blood pressure or if taking blood thinners. Raw berries may cause vomiting or diarrhea if eaten in large quantities. Otherwise, very safe.

DANDELION

Taraxacum officinale

FAMILY: Asteraceae

OTHER NAMES: *Fr.* Pissenlit

PARTS USED: Roots, leaves, flowers

CHARACTERISTICS: Leaves: cool, bitter, drying. Roots: sweet, bitter, cool

SYSTEMS AFFECTED: Liver, spleen, stomach, kidney, bladder

ACTIONS: Diuretic (esp. roots), tonic, alterative, cholagogue, laxative

RANGE: Introduced across all of Canada

Folder Pull Corner

Although it has been considered a pesky weed ever since well-groomed lawns became popular, it remains one of the most effective medicinal herbs available. Easily identified on every lawn and field early in the spring, it is a hardy perennial with a basal rosette of deeply toothed leaves above a central taproot. There are several slender hollow stalks emerging from each rosette containing a milky latex, all leafless with one composite yellow flowerhead, which opens in the morning and closes up when the sun goes down. These mature into white fluffy spheres which are actually seeds with tiny hairy parachutes attached that are easily dispersed in the wind. Harvest the leaves in the spring when they are tender; roots can be harvested in fall. They should be split longitudinally and dried for later use.

MEDICINAL USES:

Liver obstructions and stagnation, urinary tract infections, skin eruptions, arthritis, stomach pains

- General cleanser, it may help clear liver and gallbladder obstructions, help jaundice, stimulate and tonify the liver and gallbladder (particularly when there has been abuse over the years due to bad eating habits and alcohol abuse), increase bile production, aid digestion, balance digestive enzymes, encourage the elimination of toxins from the body. Acts as a mild laxative for chronic constipation, increases appetite.
- High in mineral content, great spring tonic, rich source of vitamins A and C, potassium, and calcium.
- Root may be useful in clearing obstructions from the spleen, pancreas, bladder, kidneys. Good for gallstones.
- A powerful diuretic, it can decrease high blood pressure and edema without depleting the body of potassium like many pharmaceuticals.
- Treats anemia with many nutritive minerals, purifies the blood.
- Helps alleviate joint pain, rheumatism, gout, arthritis.
- Combined with endives and chicory, the young leaves make a great cleansing salad and promote regularity.
- Root tea, taken 4–6 times a day, combined with a light diet of broths, rice, and mung beans, can benefit those with hepatitis.
- Can clear acne, inflammatory skin conditions. Also, the latex can be rubbed on the skin to remove warts.

OTHER USES:
- The flowers can be made into wine or jelly or added to salads.
- The roasted root makes a nice hot beverage.

DECOCTION: Combine 2–3 tsp. ground root with 1 cup water. Bring to a boil and simmer 10–15 minutes. Cool, drink 3 times a day. May be combined with Burdock root.

TINCTURE: Root, standard ratios, 1 tsp. per day.

COMBINATIONS:

For congestion in the liver, add Goldenseal, Celandine, or Barberry. Licorice root softens the bitterness. Burdock root helps with acne or rheumatic pain.

CAUTION: Do not use Dandelions from lawns that have been treated with chemicals.

DEVIL'S CLUB

Oplopanax horridus

FAMILY: Araliaceae

OTHER NAMES: Alaskan Ginseng, Devil's Walking Stick, *Fr.* Bois piquant

PARTS USED: Inner bark of roots and stems (preferably green)

SYSTEMS AFFECTED: Pancreas, spleen

CHARACTERISTICS: Cooling, moistening, bitter

ACTIONS: Anti-inflammatory, antirheumatic, diaphoretic, tonic, alterative, antidiabetic

RANGE: Native to British Columbia, Alberta, the Yukon, Ontario (sparse)

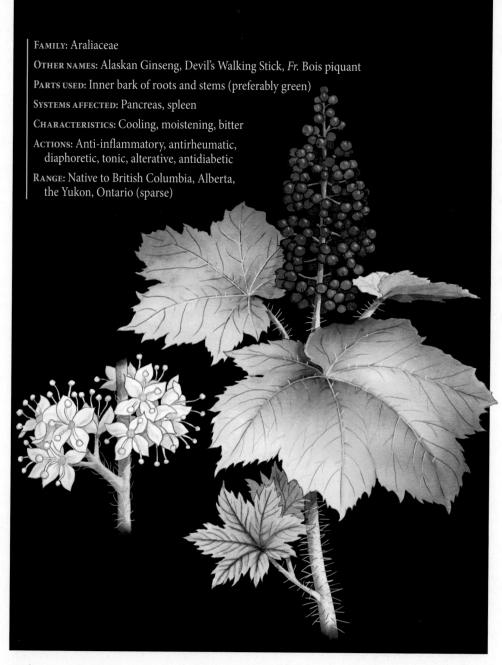

Many of the Indigenous Peoples of the Northwest Coast have traditionally considered this formidable plant sacred. Its large, maple-shaped leaves, sprawling stalks, and frightening needle-like thorns make it look almost prehistoric, growing to a height of 1 to 3 metres. Its medicine is potent and must be gathered with care and respect. A member of the Ginseng family, it has many of the same properties, affecting general health and vitality. It is usually found in old-growth forests, boggy places, and along streams and low sub-alpine elevations, the long stalks eventually falling over to root and sprout new growth, creating dense colonies. The small, fragrant, whitish-green flowers appear in the spring, growing atop a stalk in pyramid-shaped clusters, then turn to red berries in the summer. Out of respect for the importance of Devil's Club in the ceremonies and medicine of Indigenous Peoples, the risk of it becoming endangered due to clear-cutting of old-growth forests, and its slow growth rate, I don't recommend wildcrafting this plant.

MEDICINAL USES:

Arthritis, Type 2 diabetes, coughs, colds, arthritis, burnout, tuberculosis

- Recent studies show that extracts of Devil's Club root bark decrease the activity of pancreatic and intestinal enzymes, slowing the rise of glucose levels after eating a meal. This holds great promise for regulating blood sugar levels and managing Type 2 diabetes, particularly among Indigenous Peoples of the Pacific Northwest, where the plant is culturally embedded as a source for healing.
- Decoction helps soothe arthritis and rheumatism. Infused oil can be massaged into joints to relieve pain.
- Hot tea or tincture in hot water may dispel dampness from the lungs, loosen phlegm, and help speed healing. Useful for colds, flu, bronchitis, fevers.
- Antibacterial and antifungal activity, particularly in treatment of tuberculosis.
- Supports the adrenals and evens out a person's reaction to stress, helping those who have suffered burnout or trauma. On an energetic level, it helps strengthen one's boundaries (symbolized by the thorns), particularly when they are feeling invaded by negative external influences.
- May hold promise in treating some cancers, but more research is needed.
- Salve, poultices or infused oil help soothe skin irritations and sores. Infusion or tincture may also be taken to help relieve pain.
- Berries can be rubbed into the scalp to combat lice or dandruff; however, they are toxic if taken internally.

OTHER USES:
- Inner bark is chewed by shamans or hunters in many west coast First Nations during power-seeking rituals to induce a supernatural experience and protect against evil spirits. Devil's Club charcoal often mixed with red ochre and applied as a face paint.
- Early shoots edible just after sprouting.

DECOCTION: Standard ¼–½ cup up to 3 times a day

TINCTURE: Fresh 1:2, dried 1:5, in 60% alcohol. Take 15–30 drops 3 times a day.

COMBINATIONS:

Can be combined with American Ginseng for lethargy, decreased libido, and low immunity, 30 drops 3 times a day.

CAUTION: Inner bark can cause vomiting or diarrhea in large doses. Wear gloves when handling. Berries are toxic.

DOUGLAS-FIR

Pseudotsuga menziesii

FAMILY: Pinaceae

OTHER NAMES: Oregon-Pine, *Fr.* Douglas de Menzies, Sapin de Douglas

PARTS USED: Bark, needles, pitch

SYSTEMS AFFECTED: Lymphatic, immune, skin

CHARACTERISTICS: Sweet, fragrant, resinous

ACTIONS: Anti-inflammatory, astringent, antiseptic, antimicrobial, expectorant

RANGE: Native to British Columbia and Alberta

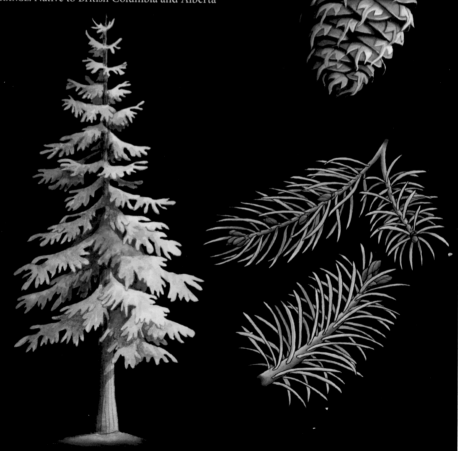

Named after the Scottish botanist David Douglas, this coniferous evergreen towers over trees of the Pacific Northwest forests, often growing up to 80 metres tall; some have been known to reach over a thousand years old. Not a true fir, its botanical name Pseudotsuga means "False Hemlock." Its needles are flat with two white stripes on the underside, and unlike true firs, they spiral around the twig. Bark of the younger trees is smooth with resin blisters, whereas the older trees' bark is ridged and furrowed. The trees are monoecious; both male and female cones grow on the same tree. The seed cones (female) can be 4–10 cm. long and hang down below the branch, turning brown before they fall to the ground. In the spring, the fresh lime-green tips of branches can be picked to make infusions, or to add a woodsy flavour to stews and soups. At certain times in the summer, some trees produce a crystalline sugar from their branch tips, which can be eaten as a confection or added to other foods as a sweetener. The bark is best harvested from thick lower branches, peeled, and dried for later use.

MEDICINAL USES:

Colds, coughs, rheumatism, excessive menstruation, kidney and bladder infection, skin inflammation, and wounds

- Astringent, an infusion of the bark will relieve diarrhea or bleeding in the intestine.
- Resin from the bark blisters is antiseptic and will heal cuts, sores, and burns and help prevent infection. It can be added to salves or oil for chest rubs for colds, congestion, or sore muscles.
- Needles and young branch tips are high in Vitamin C, and make a nice tea for colds, coughs, and asthma, or simply to quench thirst and give you energy.
- Bark infusion can slow down heavy menstrual bleeding.
- A decoction of the twigs is diuretic and tonic, helping relieve bladder or kidney complaints.
- Rheumatism and arthritis can be treated with a warm infusion compress or infused oil to ease pain and stiffness.

OTHER USES:
- Wood is strong and durable, used for fuel, building and making canoes, tepees, snowshoes; boughs used for bedding and floor coverings.
- Resin used to patch canoes or burned as incense.

INFUSION: Standard infusion or decoction, drink ½–¾ cups up to 3 times a day.

TINCTURE: Fresh 1:2, dried 1:5, in 50% alcohol. Take 15–30 drops up to 3 times a day.

COMBINATIONS:

For congestion in the liver, add Goldenseal, Celandine, or Barberry. Licorice root softens the bitterness. Burdock root helps with acne or rheumatic pain.

CAUTION: Generally safe but use in moderation.

ECHINACEA

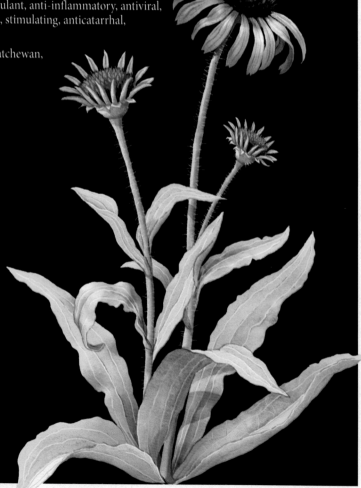

Echinacea angustifolia

FAMILY: Asteraceae

OTHER NAMES: Prairie Purple Coneflower, Narrow-leaved Purple Coneflower, *Fr.* Échinacée à feuilles étroites

PARTS USED: Whole plant

SYSTEMS AFFECTED: Lungs, immune system

CHARACTERISTICS: Sweet, diffusive (tingling), cooling, drying

ACTIONS: Immunostimulant, anti-inflammatory, antiviral, antiseptic, alterative, stimulating, anticatarrhal, lymphatic

RANGE: Native to Saskatchewan, Manitoba

Closely resembling its eastern relative, *E. purpurea*, this perennial's reputation for preventing and lessening the severity of colds and flu has become well known throughout North America. Although it had been used traditionally for at least the past four hundred years by Indigenous Peoples for treating infections and snake bites, it only rose in popularity in the seventies as an antiviral. A perennial from the Daisy family, its tall branched stems topped with striking flowers grow up to 1 metre tall and are popular as a garden flower. Echinos, Greek for "hedgehog," refers to its spiny orange-brown seedhead, which is surrounded by pink or purple petals sometimes up to 7.5 cm. long. The aerial parts contain more immune-boosting properties and are harvested in summer when the flowers emerge. The roots, although immune-enhancing as well, contain more volatile oils, and are harvested in the fall. Both are dried for later use.

MEDICINAL USES:

Respiratory tract infections, fevers, colds, flu, urinary tract infection, ear infection, Candida, skin inflammation

- Stimulates production of white blood cells, enhances the immune system, and inhibits the spread of infection. Recent clinical trials found it reduced the odds of developing a cold by 58% and decreased duration by 1–4 days. It is important to use high quality herb as soon as symptoms arise, with multiple doses taken throughout the day for the first few days, but not exceeding 10 days.
- Upper respiratory tract infections, flu, colds, sore throat, cough, fever, sinusitis, laryngitis, ear infections.
- Diffusive for strengthening and clearing lymph nodes and to clear infection from the bloodstream.
- Relieves urinary tract infections and Candida or yeast infections.
- Topically it helps heal inflammation, eczema, wounds, bites, stings, boils, poison oak, poison ivy, snake bites. May be taken internally as a root tea to increase efficacy. Reduces chance of infection.
- Root chewed to relieve toothache, reduce gum inflammation, and aid digestion.

DECOCTION: Standard decoction, ¼–½ cups up to 3 times a day.

TINCTURE: Fresh root, flowerhead, seeds, 1:2, dried 1:5, in 60% alcohol. Take 1 ml. 3–5 times a day.

CAUTION: May produce an allergic reaction in some people. Slight risk of gastrointestinal upset, rashes. May reduce the effect of medications that suppress the immune system. Consult your physician if you have an autoimmune disorder, tuberculosis, diabetes, connective tissue disorders, MS, or HIV/AIDS before using. Avoid long-term use.

ELECAMPANE

Inula helenium

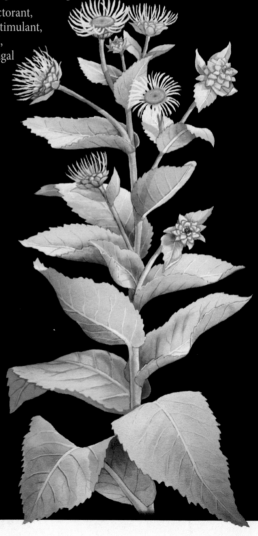

FAMILY: Asteraceae

OTHER NAMES: Horseheal, Scabwort, *Fr.* Inule aunée, Grande aunée

PARTS USED: Root, rhizome

SYSTEMS AFFECTED: Lungs, spleen, stomach

CHARACTERISTICS: Slightly bitter, sweet, pungent, warming

ACTIONS: Diuretic, tonic, diaphoretic, expectorant, alterative, antiseptic, astringent, mildly stimulant, carminative, anthelmintic, antimicrobial, antibacterial, anti-inflammatory, antifungal

RANGE: Introduced in British Columbia, Manitoba to Maritimes

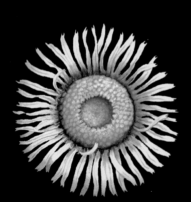

This medicinal plant is native to Europe and northwest Asia, coming over to America with the early settlers. It has since been cultivated in herb gardens, mainly for its use as an expectorant in respiratory ailments, and escaped to the wild across central and eastern North America and British Columbia. Growing from 1.2 to 1.5 metres tall, it has soft, hairy stems and large, toothed leaves, from 30 to 45 cm. long, broader at the base and pointed at the tip, with hairy undersides. The large, yellow flowers bloom all summer and resemble a shaggy, yellow daisy, about 7 to 10 cm. in diameter. Roots are gathered typically from 2- or 3-year-old plants. They have a tough, fibrous skin that can easily be peeled off, then sliced and used fresh or dried in various preparations.

MEDICINAL USES:

Respiratory tract infections, indigestion, urinary tract infections, swollen glands, tuberculosis

- The root contains up to 44% of the polysaccharide inulin, an expectorant. Chiefly used for wet coughs, it is typically used in formulas for all diseases of the lungs such as bronchitis, pneumonia, whooping cough, and asthma. Its anti-inflammatory action can soothe irritated mucous membranes and reduces mucous secretions, moving "dampness" out of the body. Although slow-acting, it has the ability to disrupt biofilms, drawing out infections that hide from antibiotics.
- Stimulates digestive function, especially in those who are often cold and tend to have constipation, soothes indigestion, relieves gas, warming and toning the digestive tract and promoting healthy gut flora. Slightly bitter, it increases bile production, and the inulin acts as a prebiotic.
- Contains sesquiterpene lactones, which may stop the growth of certain types of cancer cells.
- Has a mild influence on the lymphatic system; clears swollen glands.
- Relieves urinary tract infections and candida.
- Externally as a wash it helps heal skin inflammations.
- May eliminate parasitic worms.
- Decoction used as a mouthwash for periodontal disease and gum inflammation.

DECOCTION: Add 1 tbsp. powdered root to 2 cups water. Bring to a boil and simmer 15 minutes, then let steep for 1 hour. Take 1 tsp. 3 times a day.

TINCTURE: Fresh 1:2, dried 1:5, in 60% alcohol, 10–30 drops 4 times a day.

COUGH SYRUP: Mix ⅓ cup each of Elecampane root, Spikenard, or Sarsaparilla root, and Comfrey root. Mash and combine with 4 cups water, boil and reduce to 1 cup. Strain and add 4 tbsp. brandy and ⅔ cup honey. Take 1 tsp. every 2 hours.

COMBINATIONS:

Add Mullein and Licorice root for coughs, Aniseed and Lobelia when there are spasms and constriction in the chest.

CAUTION: Large amounts may cause vomiting, diarrhea, or cramps. Avoid if pregnant. May cause contact dermatitis in some people.

FALSE SOLOMON'S SEAL

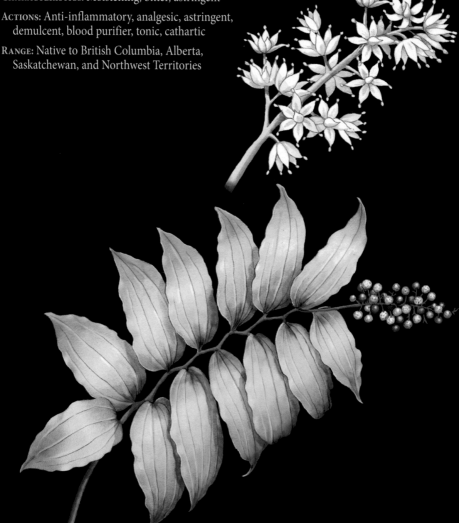

Maianthemum racemosum ssp. amplexicaule
(Smilacina racemosa)

FAMILY: Asparagaceae

OTHER NAMES: Solomon's Plume, False Spikenard, Western False Solomon's Seal, *Fr.* Smilacine à grappes

PARTS USED: Root, leaves

CHARACTERISTICS: Moistening, bitter, astringent

ACTIONS: Anti-inflammatory, analgesic, astringent, demulcent, blood purifier, tonic, cathartic

RANGE: Native to British Columbia, Alberta, Saskatchewan, and Northwest Territories

This native perennial has been used by Indigenous Peoples for centuries, but it is rarely used in modern herbal medicine. It typically grows in partial shade and in moist, soft soil in places like woodlands, shaded ravines, and streamsides. Named for its resemblance to Solomon's Seal, it usually has 7 to 12 alternate leaves growing in a similar zigzag formation; however, the flowers are very different, growing in a plume at the end of the stalk in contrast to the characteristic bell-shaped flowers that hang from the underside of the stem of Solomon's Seal. False Solomon's Seal also produces a cluster of berries that are mottled beige or green at first, turning to deep red in the fall, and although bitter raw, may be cooked and eaten in jams or jellies. They should not be confused with Solomon's Seal berries, which usually are found in pairs, and are dark blue or black and poisonous. The western subspecies amplexicaule is very similar to the eastern variety except for a more erect stem and leaves that clasp the stem. Harvest the root in the fall when foliage has died back, leaving a 7.5 cm piece with sprout in the soil for future germination.

MEDICINAL USES:

Arthritis, sore joints and ligaments, coughs, sore throat

- Decoction of root used by Indigenous Peoples to ease pain of arthritis, inflamed joints, torn ligaments, injuries, kidney issues, and back pain. It restores flexibility, lubricates and moistens connective tissue.
- Fresh root may be chewed for coughs, colds, and sore throats.
- Poultice of fresh crushed leaves or dried powdered root can be applied to wounds to stop bleeding and ease pain.
- Tea or tincture from roots used to help some menstrual disorders and regulate the cycle.
- Eases headache pain.

OTHER USES:
- Berries can be eaten in small amounts or made into jams.
- Young shoots can be picked in spring and cooked like asparagus.

DECOCTION: Standard, take ¾–1 cup up to 4 times a day.

TINCTURE: Fresh root 1:2, in 50% alcohol. Take 10–30 drops 4 times a day.

CAUTION: Berries are laxative if eaten in large amounts. Avoid if pregnant. May cause contact dermatitis in some people.

FERNLEAF BISCUITROOT

Lomatium dissectum

FAMILY: Apiaceaè

OTHER NAMES: Desert Parsley, Lomatium, Indian Parsley, Toza, *Fr.* Lomatium à feuilles découpées

PARTS USED: Root, seed

CHARACTERISTICS: Pungent, bitter, warm, drying, resinous

SYSTEMS AFFECTED: Upper respiratory, stomach

ACTIONS: Antibacterial, antiviral, antifungal, stimulating expectorant, immune stimulant

RANGE: Native to British Columbia, southern Alberta, Saskatchewan (rare)

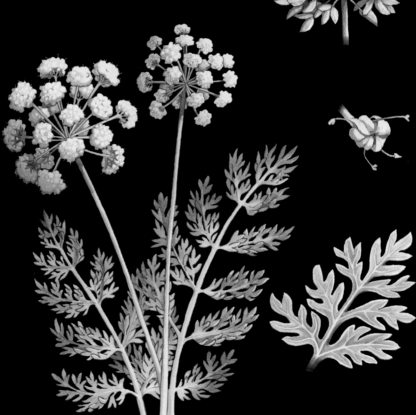

Lomatium has been highly regarded by Indigenous Peoples of the Pacific Northwest for centuries, both as food and as a potent medicine. During the pandemic of 1918–1920, an American doctor working with the Washoe people of Nevada noticed a dramatically decreased rate of infection among those who were using this herb. A native perennial of the carrot family with a long woody taproot, it is still found along the dry, rocky slopes and meadows of western Canada, although its numbers have dwindled. Its fragrant yellow or purple flowers grow in umbels of 10–30 rays atop a hollow stalk that can reach up to 1.8 metres tall. The leaves are mostly basal and divided, with fine hairs along the veins of the underside. For a time it was little used in modern herbalism; however, with the recent resurgence of new deadly viruses, interest in Lomatium has increased, some herbalists claiming it is probably our strongest and most effective antiviral herb, particularly with respiratory tract infections. The root should be at least 3 years old to be medicinally effective. Dig up in late spring or fall, slice longitudinally and hang to dry. Only take what you need, as it is becoming endangered.

MEDICINAL USES:

Respiratory tract infections, colds, flu, stomach disorders, fungal infections, sores, arthritis

- Tincture or decoction used as a powerful remedy for flus or colds, high fevers, coughs, bronchitis, pneumonia, and asthma, where the respiratory tract is involved. Dramatically reduces viral count, proven effective against many types of bacteria, mold, and fungi.
- Anecdotal evidence among herbalists has shown success in eliminating some cases of rotavirus, shingles, Epstein–Barr, cytomegalovirus, chronic fatigue, HIV, hepatitis C, candidiasis, urinary tract infection, and H1N1, although few clinical trials have been done to date.
- Decoctions of the root have been used internally to treat stomach disorders, and as a dietary tonic to help gain weight or build immunity.
- Decoctions used externally as a poultice for arthritis, sores, boils, bruises, wounds, or as a rinse for mouth or gum infections. Effective against periodontal disease. A few drops of tincture placed on a Band-Aid and kept on for 4 or 5 days may get rid of warts.

OTHER USES: Young shoots can be cooked as greens, and the root can be boiled and eaten, or dried and ground to a powder and added to flours or soups.

FOLKLORE: Some American Indigenous men used to carry the seed as a love charm.

TINCTURE: Use 3 parts Everclear alcohol to 1 part distilled water. Chop dried root finely and fill a Mason jar about ¼ full (fresh root ½ full), cover with alcohol mixture to the top and cap. Shake vigorously and store in a dark place for at least 2 weeks. Strain and bottle. Start with 5–10 drops diluted in water, once a day for a week, and increase if well tolerated, up to 30 drops 4 times a day.

CAUTION: May cause itchy rashes in a small percentage of patients taking it for the first time. To reduce likelihood of rash, take Dandelion root, and discontinue use if rash becomes severe. Safety during pregnancy unknown so not recommended.

FEVERFEW

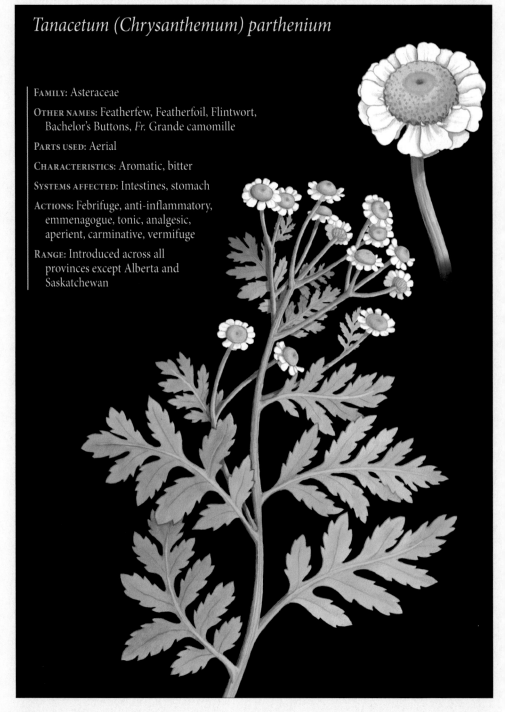

Tanacetum (Chrysanthemum) parthenium

FAMILY: Asteraceae

OTHER NAMES: Featherfew, Featherfoil, Flintwort, Bachelor's Buttons, *Fr.* Grande camomille

PARTS USED: Aerial

CHARACTERISTICS: Aromatic, bitter

SYSTEMS AFFECTED: Intestines, stomach

ACTIONS: Febrifuge, anti-inflammatory, emmenagogue, tonic, analgesic, aperient, carminative, vermifuge

RANGE: Introduced across all provinces except Alberta and Saskatchewan

This erect perennial or biennial is a European native now common throughout North America but grows mostly in gardens, occasionally escaping into the wild or remaining around old homesteads. Its branched leafy stem is furrowed, about 60 cm. high, with alternate pinnate leaves, its leaflets gashed and toothed. The compound flowers resemble a small daisy, its centre convex and bright yellow, the petals often doubled. It flowers throughout the summer and is aromatic. Bees dislike it and will keep their distance. Gather in early summer and dry for later use.

MEDICINAL USES:

Migraines, fevers, irregular menstruation, stomach upset, arthritis

- As its name suggests, Feverfew was once known for its fever-reducing properties and usefulness for the common cold, but there are other herbs that are more effective. Its main use now is in preventing and treating migraines and has been proven effective in several scientific studies where patients who took capsules of Feverfew every day had fewer migraines after 12 weeks and they were less intense. Like many herbs, a small and regular dose over a long period of time works better than a large amount over a short period of time.
- Increases appetite, improves digestion, helps relieve colic and colitis.
- May help reduce skin inflammation and relieve dermatitis.
- Uterine stimulant, promotes menstruation, eases irregularities and cramps. Tones the womb after childbirth.
- There is some promising research into using Feverfew and St. John's Wort for diabetic peripheral neuropathy.
- May relieve the pain and inflammation of arthritis and rheumatism.
- Some claim it will relieve tinnitus and Meniere's disease.

FOLKLORE: When planted around one's dwelling, was said to purify the air and prevent disease. Often used to ward off insects.

INFUSION: ½–1 tsp. dried or fresh herb to 1 cup of boiling water, cool. Take ½ cup twice a day.

TINCTURE: Standard. Take 1 ml per day.

CAUTION: Not recommended if pregnant or nursing. Avoid if you are prone to allergies. If taking for more than a week and wish to stop, reduce gradually, as stopping all at once may cause headaches, anxiety, muscle stiffness, and joint pain. May increase the risk of bleeding. Avoid if you are on blood thinners. Ask your doctor before taking if you are on any medications. Do not give to children under two years of age.

FIREWEED

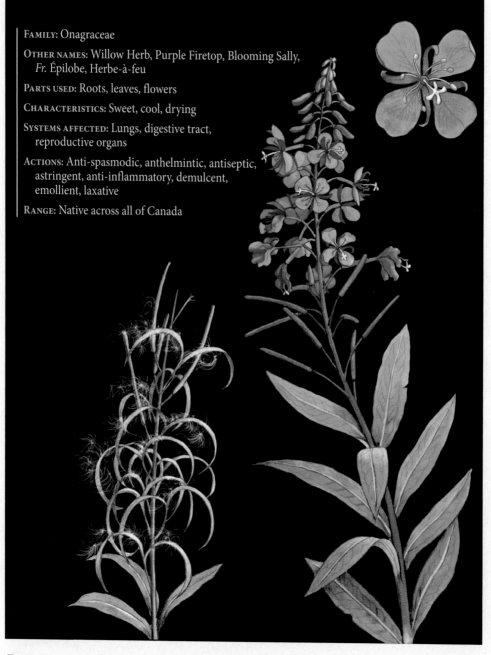

Chamaenerion (Epilobium) angustifolium

FAMILY: Onagraceae

OTHER NAMES: Willow Herb, Purple Firetop, Blooming Sally, *Fr.* Épilobe, Herbe-à-feu

PARTS USED: Roots, leaves, flowers

CHARACTERISTICS: Sweet, cool, drying

SYSTEMS AFFECTED: Lungs, digestive tract, reproductive organs

ACTIONS: Anti-spasmodic, anthelmintic, antiseptic, astringent, anti-inflammatory, demulcent, emollient, laxative

RANGE: Native across all of Canada

This colourful flower is noted for being one of the first plants to appear after a fire; it thrives on burnt or disturbed land and can become invasive very quickly as it spreads both by self-seeding and rhizomes. Native to North America, it is a perennial herb growing up to 1.8 metres tall with magenta flowers that bloom from July into September. They bloom low on the stem at first, then throughout the summer they work their way up to the top. In the fall the seedpods split open and the plant tops become white and feathery, the tufts of white hair distributing the seeds on the wind. The willow-like alternate leaves are dark green above and silvery underneath with a lighter central vein. The lateral veins are unique, as they don't extend to the outer edge but loop together near the margin. Young shoots may be picked in the spring and eaten fresh in salads. Leaves can be picked early in the summer and dried in a paper bag, then stored in a glass jar for later use. The root should be dug in the fall and may be used fresh, mashed as a poultice for inflammations.

MEDICINAL USES:

Asthma, coughs, irritable bowel, diarrhea, skin problems

- Whole plant is edible and is a gentle but effective anti-inflammatory. Rich in Vitamin C, calcium and iron. Tannins tighten tissues and dry out "dampness" or mucous production.
- Antispasmodic, demulcent, high in mucilage, soothes mucous membranes; cool decoction of the whole plant used to treat whooping cough, asthma, hiccups.
- Leaf decoctions are anti-inflammatory and good for the stomach and the digestive tract, soothe and rebalance irritable bowel and diarrhea. Especially good for summer bowel complaints.
- Young flowerheads may be infused in oil for treating hemorrhoids.
- Indigenous Peoples traditionally use the peeled root in poultices for boils or abscesses and the leaves in compresses soothe burns, psoriasis, eczema, acne, and wounds, and speed healing. Also used as a tea for digestive and bronchial problems.
- Current research shows the rhizome, which contains flavonoids and the tannin oenothein B, may be useful in treating benign prostatic hyperplasia and possibly prostate cancer.

OTHER USES:
- Young shoots and flowers are good in salads or as a potherb.
- Dried leaves make a nice tea.
- Yields a delicious honey.
- Cordage made from fibrous stems.
- Cottony seed hairs can be used as stuffing or tinder.

INFUSION: 1–2 tsp. dried herb in 1 cup of boiling water. Drink as needed.

IVAN CHAI (FERMENTED) TEA: Collect stalks before or during flowering. Remove leaves and allow to wilt for about 12–18 hours on a sheet of cloth. Take 4 or 5 leaves at a time and roll together between the palms to bruise, then place loosely into a bowl and cover with a lid or plate, stirring often to aerate. When they become fragrant and dark in colour, stop the fermentation process (usually 3–5 days). Place in oven at lowest temperature setting until completely dry. Store in airtight container.

CAUTION: Do not use during the early stages of pregnancy, as it is a uterine stimulant and could cause miscarriage. Do not exceed recommended dose. Avoid use 2 weeks before or after surgery.

FULLER'S TEASEL

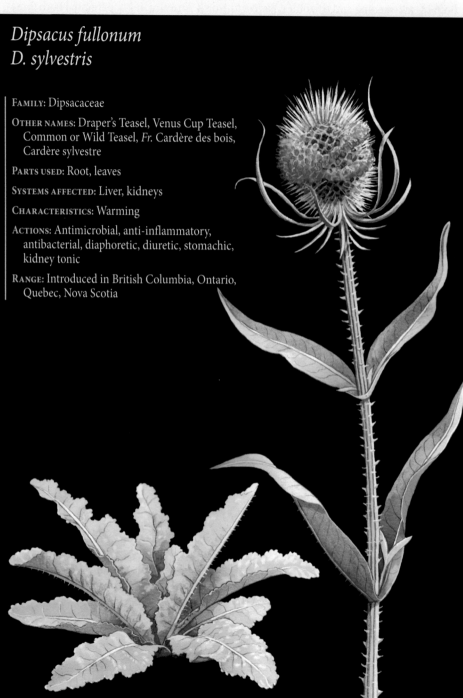

Dipsacus fullonum
D. sylvestris

FAMILY: Dipsacaceae

OTHER NAMES: Draper's Teasel, Venus Cup Teasel, Common or Wild Teasel, *Fr.* Cardère des bois, Cardère sylvestre

PARTS USED: Root, leaves

SYSTEMS AFFECTED: Liver, kidneys

CHARACTERISTICS: Warming

ACTIONS: Antimicrobial, anti-inflammatory, antibacterial, diaphoretic, diuretic, stomachic, kidney tonic

RANGE: Introduced in British Columbia, Ontario, Quebec, Nova Scotia

There is little history of use of Teasel in Western herbal medicine, but it has recently gained popularity for its potential effectiveness in treating Lyme Disease. A native of Europe/Eurasia, it was introduced to North America, usually growing in ditches, fields, and waste places throughout British Columbia and Central and Eastern Canada. Sometimes growing up to 1.8 metres tall, it is easily recognized by its spiky oval flowerhead with rings of mauve-coloured blooms and long spiny bracts. A biennial plant, its first year of growth consists of a rosette of prickly basal leaves and a taproot that can extend 60 cm. or more into the ground. In the second year, a prickly stem emerges, with erect branches terminated by the flowerhead. The lance-shaped opposite leaves may measure up to 30 cm. long and have toothed or wavy edges and spines along the central vein. The flowerhead turns brown in the fall but the stem remains stiff throughout the winter and is often used in dried flower arrangements. The roots are best harvested before the flower stem emerges in the second year, between fall and spring, and tinctured fresh.

MEDICINAL USES:

Lyme disease, arthritis, stiff and painful joints and muscles, lack of appetite, acne, warts

- Has been shown to be effective in treating Lyme disease. After treatments with antibiotics, sometimes symptoms remain, as the bacteria causing it will often hide in the body's tissues and continue reinfecting the patient for months or years after treatment. Teasel is able to coax them out into the bloodstream, where the immune system is able to tackle them more effectively.
- Diuretic and diaphoretic action helps rid the body of toxins and reduces intermittent fevers.
- Tonifies the liver and kidneys, improves circulation, and treats jaundice.
- Strengthens connective tissue, eases pain in the joints and lower back, reduces arthritic pain and stiffness. Helps chronic inflammation and soothes nerve pain.
- Infusion strengthens the stomach, improves the appetite.
- Infusion of the leaves applied externally can help acne.
- Ointment made from the roots has been used to remove warts.

OTHER USES:
- Blue dye obtained from the dried plant.
- Early wool manufacturers attached the dried seed heads to a spindle to comb, or tease, the wool to raise the nap.

TINCTURE (FOR LYME DISEASE OR PAIN): Fresh roots 1:2 in 50% alcohol. Start with only one drop 3 times per day, adding one more drop daily until symptoms subside.

CAUTION: Rash may develop with use; reduce dosage if this occurs. May react with anti-inflammatory drugs and antidepressants. Avoid if pregnant or breastfeeding due to lack of research.

GHOST PIPES

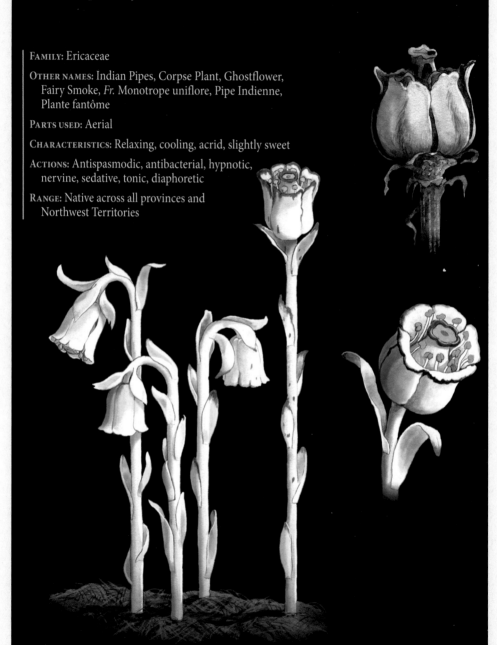

Monotropa uniflora

FAMILY: Ericaceae

OTHER NAMES: Indian Pipes, Corpse Plant, Ghostflower, Fairy Smoke, *Fr.* Monotrope uniflore, Pipe Indienne, Plante fantôme

PARTS USED: Aerial

CHARACTERISTICS: Relaxing, cooling, acrid, slightly sweet

ACTIONS: Antispasmodic, antibacterial, hypnotic, nervine, sedative, tonic, diaphoretic

RANGE: Native across all provinces and Northwest Territories

This strange, ghostly perennial is typically found growing in clumps under trees in moist, shaded forests across North America. Reaching a height of 10–30 cm., its unique white colour is due to its lack of chlorophyll. It depends instead on a parasitic relationship with the mycelial networks or fungi below the surface for its nutrients. These fungi, which grow amongst the fine roots and rhizomes of the neighbouring trees, pull water and minerals from the soil, which are then taken in by the tree, pulling them up the trunk to nourish the leaves so photosynthesis can occur. The sugars created then flow back down the trunk to the roots, where they are absorbed by the mycelium, creating a symbiotic network where each communicates and feeds off the other. Ghost Pipes tap into the nodes connecting the tree roots to the fungus, drawing nutrients from both. The mass of roots sends up several white, waxy stalks with scale-like leaves that turn black when touched, and terminates in a solitary flower, which curves downward. As it matures, the flower turns up, the plant turns black or brown, and its seedpod dries out, releasing tiny seeds over the forest floor. Pick only the aerial parts, as the roots will produce more plants if not disturbed, and only take a small percentage, as these plants are becoming rare.

In recent years, the safety of Ghost Pipes has come into question and become a topic of debate between herbalists due to the presence of grayanotoxin, a neurotoxin also found in Rhododendron and Mountain Laurel. Although there is very little research on this subject, it is safer to stay away from using it internally until more information is made available.

MEDICINAL USES:

Seizures, anxiety, panic attacks, spasms, toothache, eye inflammation, chronic pain

- Long history of use by Indigenous Peoples; an infusion can be used as a remedy for convulsions, panic attacks, anxiety, fainting, or any condition where there is emotional or sensory overload. Relieves spasms and calms the nervous system.
- Has a mild analgesic action on pain, but it's more useful at helping deal with chronic or acute pain by reducing sensitivity to it without being completely overwhelming. It eases emotional pain by helping people detach from it so they can deal with it more effectively. Can bring people down from a bad drug-induced experience, helping them feel more grounded.
- Infusion can be used for colds and to bring down a fever.
- Crushed plant can be rubbed on bunions or warts, poultice used on sores that are taking a long time to heal.
- Flowers chewed for toothaches.
- Juice of the plant mixed with rosewater can be ingested to soothe bladder inflammation and ulcers. It can also be applied to the eyes with a sterile cloth to ease conjunctivitis, pinkeye, or inflammation.

CAUTION: Internal use not recommended. Contains glycosides, and may be poisonous if eaten in large doses. May cause vivid dreams.

GOLDENROD

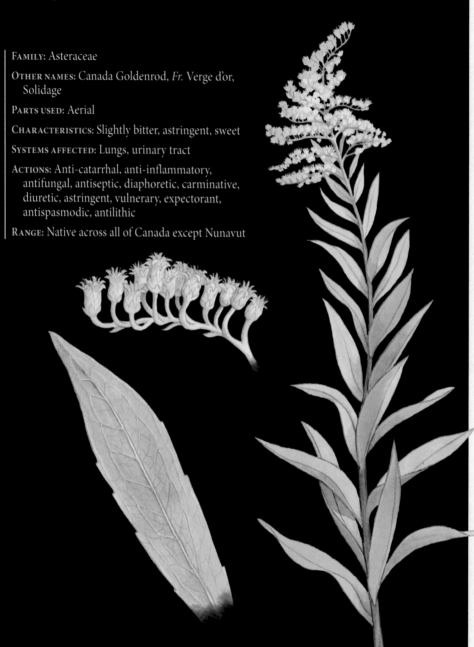

Solidago canadensis

FAMILY: Asteraceae

OTHER NAMES: Canada Goldenrod, *Fr.* Verge d'or, Solidage

PARTS USED: Aerial

CHARACTERISTICS: Slightly bitter, astringent, sweet

SYSTEMS AFFECTED: Lungs, urinary tract

ACTIONS: Anti-catarrhal, anti-inflammatory, antifungal, antiseptic, diaphoretic, carminative, diuretic, astringent, vulnerary, expectorant, antispasmodic, antilithic

RANGE: Native across all of Canada except Nunavut

Solidago, meaning "to make whole," refers to Goldenrod's ability to restore the body to health and wholeness. There are over a hundred different species across North America, *S. canadensis* being one of the native ones, used for centuries by Indigenous Peoples as a wound herb. Goldenrod grows in many different habitats, depending on the species; some prefer dry fields, others wetlands or marshes. It is a perennial with erect, often downy stems, branching at the top. The leaves are alternate, elliptical, toothed, and stalked, the upper ones smaller. There are clusters of small, yellow flowers; the European variety, *S. virgaurea*, has blooms all around the stem, the Canadian variety on only one side. Harvest top third of the plant when there are buds and open flowers, but avoid plants that have wilted flowers. Pick only the top third of the plant, then hang to dry in the shade.

MEDICINAL USES:

Urinary tract infections and stones, upper respiratory problems, sore throat, skin inflammations, stomach upset, candida

- Astringent, diuretic, and anti-inflammatory, it is useful in the treatment of urinary tract infections and kidney inflammations (nephritis) and helps dissolve kidney and gallstones.
- An effective expectorant, it expels mucous and works on the upper respiratory system, soothing coughs, acute or chronic bronchitis, and asthma.
- A good source of rutin, a powerful flavonoid that increases the strength of capillaries and improves the tone of the cardiovascular system.
- Infusion may be used as a gargle for sore throats or laryngitis.
- Used for centuries as a wound herb, it is effective in poultices, ointments, and baths for treating slow-healing wounds, burns, eczema, and varicose veins.
- Soothes upset stomach, flatulence, colic.
- Tincture may be used to desensitize from seasonal allergies like ragweed.
- Prevents and treats urogenital disorders like yeast infections; infusion may be drunk as a tea or used as a douche.

OTHER USES: Flowers produce a strong yellow dye.

INFUSION: 1 tbsp. fresh or 2–3 tsp. dried herb, infused in 1 cup boiling water for 10–15 minutes. Mint or honey may also be added. Drink 3 times a day. May increase urination or coughing/sneezing when you first start using it.

COMBINATIONS:

Works well with Bearberry or Elderflower for urinary problems. Combine with Thyme or Mullein for upper respiratory infections.

CAUTION: Avoid use if pregnant or breastfeeding, have hyper- or hypotension, heart or kidney disease, or are allergic to Goldenrod. May interact with some medications; consult a professional before use.

HAIRY ARNICA

Arnica mollis

FAMILY: Asteraceae

OTHER NAMES: *Fr.* Arnica douce, Arnica moelleux

PARTS USED: Flowerheads

CHARACTERISTICS: Warm, drying

SYSTEMS AFFECTED: Blood, circulation

ACTIONS: Stimulant, analgesic, anticoagulant, nervine, vasodilator, anti-inflammatory, vulnerary

RANGE: Native to British Columbia, Alberta, the Yukon, Northwest Territories, Quebec

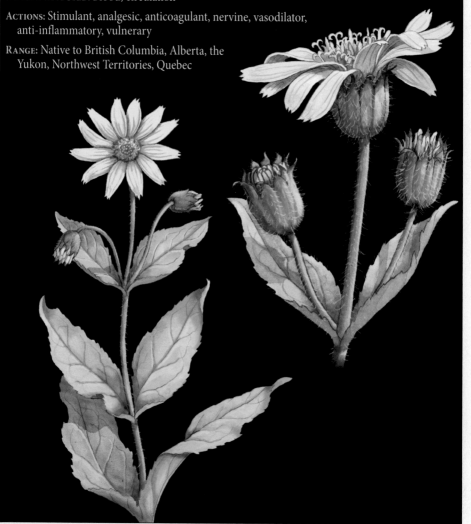

Similar to the European variety *Arnica montana*, Arnica grows all across Canada, but this species is mostly found in subalpine meadows, fields, and foothills of Western Canada, spreading in thick mats by underground rhizomes. As its name suggests, most of the plant is hairy. The erect stem grows from 15 to 61 cm. tall and has 2–4 pairs of opposite leaves, which can be up to 18 cm. long and are irregularly toothed and lance-shaped. Basal leaves are smaller and elliptical, and may be on separate shoots. The bright yellow composite flowers appear throughout the summer, with 12–20 petals that are grooved lengthwise and toothed at the tip. Typically one flower emerges at the top, followed by two others below on shorter stems. Gather only the flowerheads, preferably just after opening, and dry for later use.

MEDICINAL USES:

Sprains, swellings, bruises, sore muscles, soft tissue injuries

- Infused oil, salve, or gel rubbed on the skin relieves sore, aching muscles, bruising, sprains, joint inflammation, arthritis, bunions. Stimulates the white blood cells to remove congested blood and debris around injury sites and inflamed tissue. If rubbed on immediately after injuring, a bruise might not even appear. Do not use if skin is broken.
- Can ease symptoms of carpal tunnel syndrome.
- Reduces swelling from insect bites, bone fractures.

INFUSED OIL: Fill a Mason jar ⅔ full with dried flower petals. Cover with olive oil, seal, and place in a dark place and let macerate 4–6 weeks. Strain through several layers of cheesecloth, bottle and label.

POULTICE: Place a handful of flowerheads into boiling water, cover, and let steep until it has reached room temperature. Wrap flowers in cheesecloth and apply to skin to relieve bruising, arthritis, or inflammation.

CAUTION: Toxic if taken internally. Stomach irritation may occur if used internally. High doses may cause dizziness, tremors, tachycardia, arrhythmia, and collapse. Do not use on broken skin.

HAWTHORN

Crataegus monogyna
C. douglasii (Black Hawthorn)

FAMILY: Rosaceae

OTHER NAMES: *C. monogyna*: One-seeded Hawthorn, English Hawthorn, May Thorn, White Thorn, *Fr.* Aubépine; *C. douglasii*: Black Hawthorn, River Hawthorn, Columbia Hawthorn, *Fr.* Aubépine noire

PARTS USED: Leaves, flowering tips of branches, berries, bark

SYSTEMS AFFECTED: Heart, upper GI tract

CHARACTERISTICS: Sour, slightly warm, sweet (berries); cool, astringent (flowering tips)

ACTIONS: Anti-inflammatory, antioxidant, antihypertensive, adaptogen, cardiotonic, diuretic, astringent

RANGE: *C. monogyna* introduced in British Columbia, Ontario, Quebec, Maritimes; *C. douglasii* native to British Columbia, Alberta, Saskatchewan, Ontario

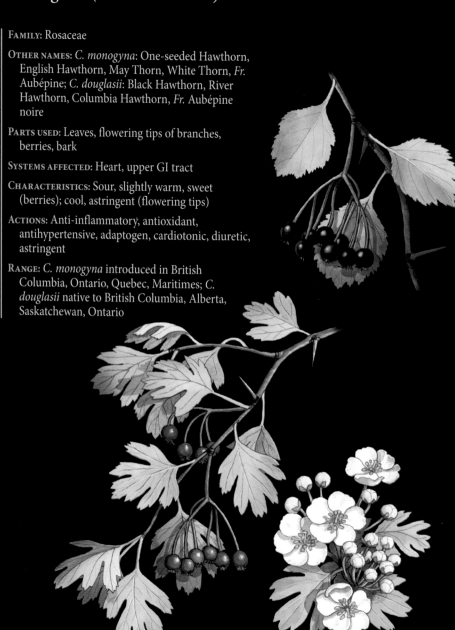

This deciduous shrub or small tree from the rose family has been a favoured heart remedy in Europe for centuries. There are over 100 species in North America, however *C. monogyna*, and occasionally our native *C. douglasii* are the ones most often used for medicines. Their thorny branches and pretty white flowers make them ideal for hedgerows if you wish to keep out unwanted visitors. English Hawthorn grows up to 10 metres tall, it has alternate toothed leaves with 3–7 lobes and thorns about 1.3 cm. long. The white or pink flowers usually emerge in May, giving off a slight fishy odour which attracts pollinators then fades when the flowers are dried. Black Hawthorn is slightly smaller, its leaves are not lobed and are finely toothed, and the "haws," or berries, are black when fully ripe. The branch tips and flowers can be hung upside down or placed in a paper bag until crisp. The haws are gathered in late August or September and can be dried for later use. Both can be tinctured fresh if desired.

MEDICINAL USES:

High blood pressure, angina, atherosclerosis, high cholesterol, digestive problems, poor circulation, anxiety

- Contains flavonoids, which reduce inflammation and cause dilation of the smooth muscles lining the coronary arteries, subsequently increasing blood flow to the heart. This makes heart contractions more efficient, bringing more oxygen and nutrients into the heart cells and reducing conditions like angina, early stages of congestive heart failure, and mild arrhythmia. Antioxidants help to strengthen blood vessels, making arterial walls more pliable. In human clinical trials with people who have had chronic heart failure, it was shown to improve exercise tolerance and reduce fatigue and shortness of breath when taken for 3–16 weeks with only mild adverse effects. Slow acting and nourishing, it should be taken for at least 3 months to see an effect.
- Fruit extract soothes digestive problems, helping to break down fats and providing fibre and probiotic action to improve transit time. Helps relieve stomach ulcers. Astringency helps settle diarrhea and irritation in the gut.
- Improves circulation to the extremities.
- May reduce anxiety, bring a sense of calm to stressful situations.
- Berries high in Vitamin C.

OTHER USES:
- Used to make jams, jellies, candy, wine, or cordial.
- Europeans used it for spiritual protection and to decorate the maypole, a pagan symbol of renewal and fertility.

TINCTURE: Fresh leaves, flowers 1:2, dried plant and/or berries 1:5, in 60% alcohol. Take 10–30 drops up to 3 times a day. Should be continued for at least 4 months to get maximum benefit.

INFUSION: Steep 1–2 tsp. leaves and flowers 15–30 min. in boiling water. Drink up to 3 cups a day. Cold infusion of berries, 2–4 tbsp. up to twice a day.

CAUTION: May interfere with digoxin or other heart medications. Consult doctor before use. May cause vertigo, dizziness, mild nausea, agitation.

HEAL-ALL

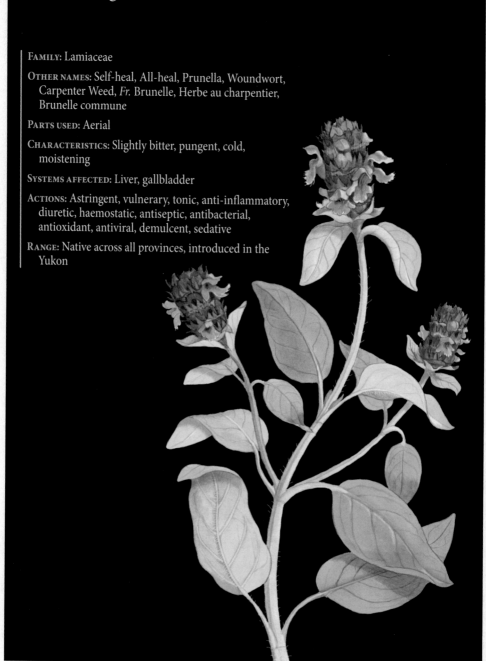

Prunella vulgaris

FAMILY: Lamiaceae

OTHER NAMES: Self-heal, All-heal, Prunella, Woundwort, Carpenter Weed, *Fr.* Brunelle, Herbe au charpentier, Brunelle commune

PARTS USED: Aerial

CHARACTERISTICS: Slightly bitter, pungent, cold, moistening

SYSTEMS AFFECTED: Liver, gallbladder

ACTIONS: Astringent, vulnerary, tonic, anti-inflammatory, diuretic, haemostatic, antiseptic, antibacterial, antioxidant, antiviral, demulcent, sedative

RANGE: Native across all provinces, introduced in the Yukon

Although this native perennial herb of the Mint family was once used, as its name suggests, to heal just about anything, it has somewhat lost its popularity with herbalists over the years, but new research suggests it could prove to be quite useful. It grows up to 30 cm. high, and is easily identified by its dense cluster of purple flowers at the top of a square stem. They grow in rings around the fat cylindrical spike, looking somewhat ragged since they are never all in bloom at once, and each tubular flower is composed of a two-lipped calyx with dark red tips and a two-lipped purple corolla resembling a throat. Below the flower spike is a set of two stalkless leaves and then more paired opposite leaves on stems branching off of a creeping stem, which sends roots into the soil at intervals. It grows in fields and waste places, and can be picked in the summer or fall and dried for later use.

MEDICINAL USES:

Wounds, sore throat, swollen lymph nodes, hemorrhoids

- High in antioxidants and antiseptic, a lukewarm infusion makes a nourishing drink, or mixed with honey can be used as a gargle for sore throats and mouth infections. Enhances the immune system, works well with the lymphatic system to reduce swelling as in mumps, swollen glands, and mastitis. Weak infusion may be used in a sterile eyewash for dry, painful eyes or conjunctivitis.
- Before the Second World War it was used extensively to clean wounds and stop hemorrhaging; the fresh leaf can be used as a poultice or in a compress. Soothes inflamed wounds or sores.
- Used internally for diarrhea, colitis, hemorrhoids, or internal bleeding.
- May be infused in oil and made into lotions or ointments for hemorrhoids, burns, skin ulcers, boils, eczema, and other skin irritations.
- Used as a spring tonic, may be eaten in salads or used as a pot herb.
- Popular in Asia, it is used in Chinese medicine for "liver heat" and to improve circulation and lower blood pressure, as well as for sore throats, wounds, and as a diuretic for kidney complaints.
- New studies show it could possibly be promising in treating herpes, HIV, breast cancer, and may provide protection from sun damage due to UVA and UVB rays.
- Some claim it may be useful in normalizing thyroid issues.

FOLKLORE: Once believed to be a holy herb and that it could drive away the devil.

INFUSION: Infuse 1–2 tsp. dried herb in 1 cup boiling water. Steep 1 hour. Drink 3 times a day or use as a gargle or lotion.

HORSETAIL

Equisetum arvense

FAMILY: Equisetaceae

OTHER NAMES: Field horsetail, Bottlebrush, Pewter Wort, Scouring Rush, *Fr.* Prêle des champs, Queue de renard

PARTS USED: Green sterile stalk

CHARACTERISTICS: Cool, dry, slightly bitter

SYSTEMS AFFECTED: Genito-urinary, kidney, skeletal

ACTIONS: Antibiotic, diuretic, astringent, vulnerary

RANGE: Native across all of Canada

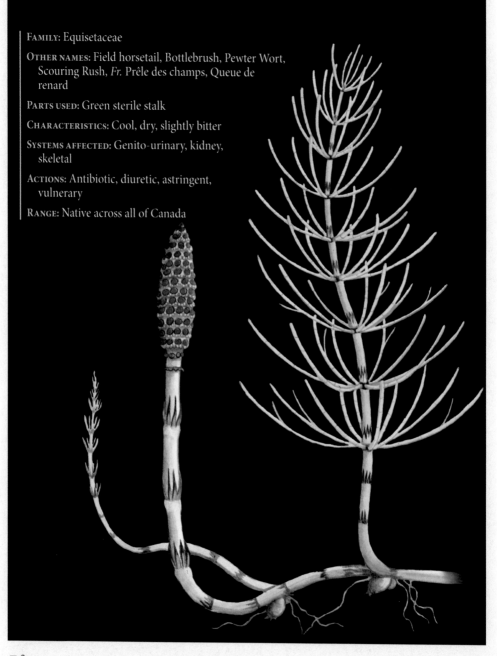

Horsetail is a rather odd-looking, prehistoric-like, non-flowering native plant that reproduces by spores located under the scales of the edible, asparagus-like shoots, a spike of around 20 cm. tall which appears in the spring. In summer the spike disappears and is replaced by a green sterile stalk that is used as medicine, with whorls of thin branches, resembling a smaller version of the large tree-like plants that covered the earth 400 million years ago. These stems and branches contain silicon crystals which also makes it useful for cleaning and polishing metal objects and kitchen utensils. It is usually found in swamps, damp woods, and fields. Gather in spring or early summer, bundle together, and hang to dry where there is good airflow.

MEDICINAL USES:

Urinary tract infections, osteoporosis, joint problems, wounds, kidney and bladder disorders

- Traditionally used as a diuretic to increase urine output and relieve chronic urinary tract infections and kidney complaints. Helps incontinence and bedwetting.
- Astringent, tightens and tones tissue in cases of diarrhea, hemorrhoids, and dysentery.
- Crushed sterile stems used as a poultice will stop bleeding and heal cuts, sores, and other wounds. Astringent, it stops hemorrhaging.
- Reduces inflammation of the prostate.
- Because of the presence of silica, a mineral essential to bone health, it strengthens and heals joints and bones. It has been suggested that it may be used as a treatment for osteoporosis, however, there is no scientific evidence yet.
- Dissolved in the bath, it can be soothing for rheumatic pain, rashes or other wounds. In a foot bath it can ease infections.
- Liquid obtained from boiling stems often used as a mouthwash or gargle for oral infections, cankers, or sore throats. Add salt if desired.
- A few drops of tincture mixed with coconut oil used topically helps keeps hair shiny, strengthens brittle nails, and prevents aging of the skin.

OTHER USES:
- As an abrasive for scouring pots and pans or polishing metal.
- Can be used as a plant spray to reduce the influence of problematic fungi in the environment. Simply steep in boiling water for an hour, strain, and cool before spraying on your plant's leaves.

BATH SOAK: Steep 1 cup of horsetail in hot water for 1 hour. Add liquid to bath water.

COMPRESS: Crush dried herb and soak in enough warm water to make a paste. Mix with crushed plantain if desired. Apply to boils or other sores twice a day.

INFUSION: 2 tsp. dried plant infused in 1 cup boiling water for 15 minutes. Strain. Drink 3 times a day. This can be mixed with lemon juice and salt to be used as a gargle.

COMBINATIONS:

Goes well with Red Clover, Stinging Nettles, and Peppermint.

CAUTION: Avoid internal use for more than a week at a time or in large quantities. Green stalks should not be eaten raw. Do not use if you are diabetic or have a deficiency in thiamine or potassium as its diuretic properties may remove these nutrients. Avoid if pregnant or nursing.

JUNIPER

Juniperus communis (Common)
J. horizontalis (Creeping)

FAMILY: Cupressaceae

OTHER NAMES: *Fr.* Genévrier

PARTS USED: Berries (cones), needles

SYSTEMS AFFECTED: Urinary, digestive

CHARACTERISTICS: Warming, spicy, pungent, drying

ACTIONS: Antibacterial, alterative, aromatic, carminative, diaphoretic, diuretic, stomachic, tonic

RANGE: Native across all of Canada

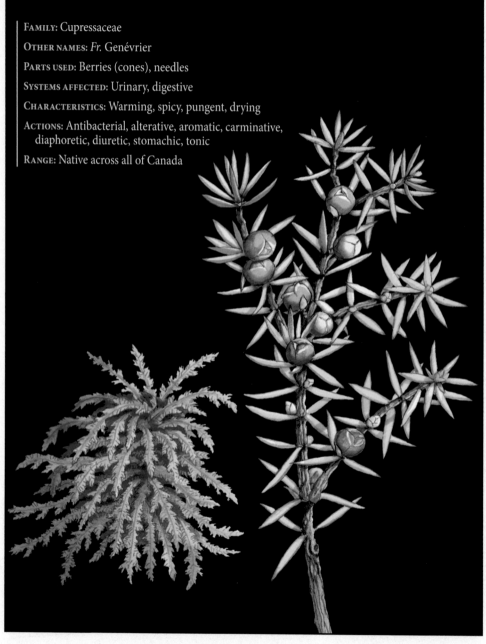

This coniferous evergreen is one of the most widely distributed across the world, including sixty species just in the Northern Hemisphere. In Canada, they grow mostly as shrubs from 0.9–1.2 metres in height, although they have been known to reach 9 metres. Its use as a purifying herb began with the ancient Greeks and continued in Europe where it was highly regarded as a kidney tonic. The Egyptians also used it in their mummification process. The Common variety usually used medicinally has needle-like leaves that grow in whorls of three around the branch, and unlike other varieties such as Creeping Juniper, they do not become scale-like as they mature. The bark is reddish-brown and peels off in thin, vertical strips. Its resinous, fragrant berries, the part primarily used as medicine, are actually female cones that take three years to mature, turning a dark blue with a powdery coating when ready to harvest, usually in the fall. They can be eaten raw, tasting a bit like gin, or they can be dried and ground as flavouring or medicine.

MEDICINAL USES:

Urinary tract infections, liver stagnation, digestive problems, diabetes, gout, menstrual cramps, colds and flu, coughs, burns

- Berries are a powerful diuretic; clear bladder and kidneys of excess uric acid, cleanse and strengthen the kidneys, relieve gout, prostatitis.
- Useful when there is "dampness" and congestion, with a coating on the tongue. Warms and dries up mucous as in colds, flu, and sinus infection and bronchitis. Helps relieve coughs and clears phlegm, strengthens immunity.
- Aids sluggish digestion, expels gas, relieves heartburn, stimulates appetite. Where there is stagnation, it will stimulate the liver and gallbladder.
- Increases contractions during childbirth, helps relieve cramps and PMS.
- Externally, a poultice of leaves pounded to a paste may be applied to burns or boils, or to ease toothaches or sore gums.
- Dried berries are astringent, decoction may be used to clear acne, eczema, dandruff. Diluted essential oil rubbed on the skin warms and soothes arthritic joints.
- Testing with Chinese Juniper berries has shown it may have antidiabetic properties, lowering blood sugar levels in rats, but more research is needed on humans.

OTHER USES:
- Added to cooking meats, stews, sauerkraut, soups.
- Burned as smudge in Indigenous ceremonies to cleanse a space of negative energies.
- The Dutch use the berries to flavour their gin.
- A bush planted near the front door was once believed to repel witches.

INFUSION: Steep ½–1 tsp. powdered berries in 1 cup boiled water, covered, for 30 minutes. Strain and drink ½ cup 2–3 times a day

TINCTURE: Dried berries 1:5, in 75% alcohol. Take 15–40 drops per day.

COMBINATIONS:

For coughs and colds, may be combined with demulcents like Coltsfoot, Slippery Elm, or Marshmallow to reduce irritation of the kidneys.

CAUTION: Can be irritating to the kidneys. Consult a professional if you have kidney problems. Avoid if pregnant or breastfeeding. Not for use by children. Use only ripe berries. Essential oil can cause blistering if undiluted. Not recommended for long-term use.

LABRADOR TEA

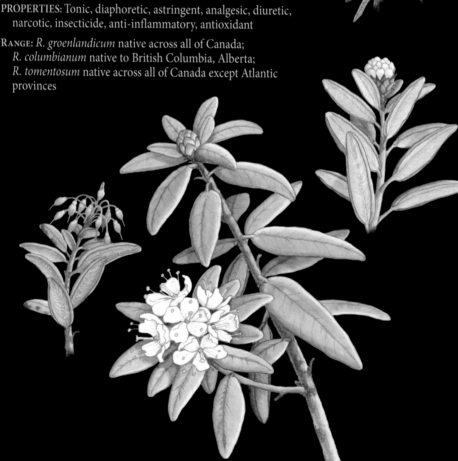

Rhododendron (Ledum) groenlandicum
R. columbianum (glandulosum) (Western)
R. tomentosum (palustre) (Northern)

FAMILY: Ericaceae

OTHER NAMES: Bog Labrador Tea, Muskeg Tea, *Fr.* Thé du Labrador, Lédon de Groenland

PARTS USED: Leaves, flowers

CHARACTERISTICS: Spicy, fragrant

SYSTEMS AFFECTED: Kidneys, liver

PROPERTIES: Tonic, diaphoretic, astringent, analgesic, diuretic, narcotic, insecticide, anti-inflammatory, antioxidant

RANGE: *R. groenlandicum* native across all of Canada; *R. columbianum* native to British Columbia, Alberta; *R. tomentosum* native across all of Canada except Atlantic provinces

Labrador Tea is a native evergreen shrub that has long been used, both by Indigenous Peoples as a soothing tea and medicine, and by European settlers as a tea replacement during shortages throughout North America. It grows in bogs, moist forests, and along roadsides to a height of up to 1.5–2 metres, with alternate elliptical leaves that are green and leathery on top and rusty coloured and woolly underneath. They droop slightly on the branch and their edges are rolled under. In June and July there are tiny clusters of white flowers that form on the end of each hairy stalk. The leaves are best if collected in the spring just before the flowers open.

MEDICINAL PROPERTIES

Respiratory infections, skin irritations, diabetes, headaches, kidney ailments

- Fragrant and soothing tea used for centuries by many northern Indigenous Peoples. An infusion of the leaves is used to treat stomach flu, diarrhea, headaches, arthritis, muscle pain, urinary tract infections, and to facilitate childbirth. A poultice or strong decoction may be used for burns, scalds, or to stop bleeding. Powdered leaves may be used for rashes and skin irritations.
- Indigenous Peoples use the tea to treat kidney ailments and stones and as a tonic and blood purifier. The Cree use it as an anti-diabetic medicine, as it has been shown to lower blood glucose levels and improve insulin levels.
- Studies show *R. tomentosum* may be effective in treating acute myeloid leukemia using a variety of solvents to maximize extraction of ursolic acid and quercetin, believed to be responsible for its anti-AML activity. However, more studies are needed.

OTHER USES:
- Leaves strewn in closets keep moths away.
- Tincture used to kill lice, mosquitoes, and fleas, repels mice.
- Brown dye obtained from plant.
- Used as flavouring in stews and marinades.

INFUSION: Put 2 tsp. herb into a pot and cover with 4 cups of water. Bring to a boil until the water turns light green. Strain out water and add another 4 cups to the pot, bringing it back to a boil. When the water turns yellow, strain into a teapot; drink no more than 2 cups per day.

CAUTION: Do not boil tea if using internally. Brew for only a short period of time in an open container. Contains ledol, a poisonous terpene which may cause headaches, cramping, or paralysis in high doses. Not recommended for pregnant or lactating women. Do not consume in excess as it is slightly narcotic.

LARCH

Larix occidentalis
L. laricina

FAMILY: Pinaceae

OTHER NAMES: *L. occidentalis*: Western Larch, *Fr.* Mélèze de l'Ouest; *L. laricina*: Tamarack, Eastern Larch, Black Larch, Hackmatack, *Fr.* Mélèze Laricin

PARTS USED: Resin, needles, bark, wood

SYSTEMS AFFECTED: Digestive, immune, respiratory

ACTIONS: Alterative, antiseptic, anti-inflammatory, diuretic, expectorant, immune stimulant, laxative, vulnerary

RANGE: *L. occidentalis* native to British Columbia, Alberta; *L. laricina* native across all of Canada

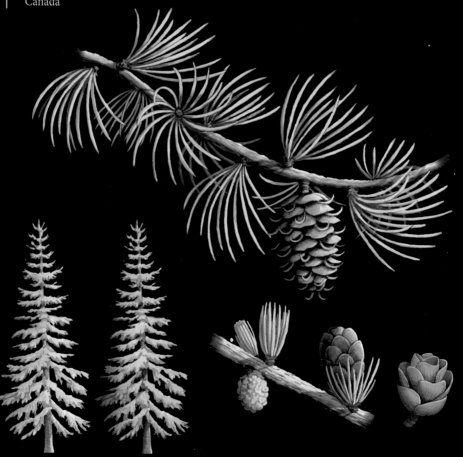

O ften called Hackmatack, derived from the Algonquin word akemantak, meaning "wood used for snowshoes," this tree is a deciduous conifer. Where other conifers remain green and keep their needles all year round, Larches turn bright yellow in the fall and lose their needles over the winter. They grow to a height of 20–60 metres depending on the species, and prefer sun and moist soil, tolerating cold temperatures. Western Larch, the largest of the Larches, grows in the mountainous regions of western Canada. It is very fire-tolerant, its bark resistant to sparks. It often sheds its lower branches as it matures, and it can live for hundreds of years. Its needles are flat on top and ridged beneath, growing in clusters along the branch. Female cones grow above the male cones and vary between red and purple when young, appearing from May to July and maturing in the fall. Fresh green tips are best gathered in early spring.

MEDICINAL USES:

Wounds, coughs, colds, irritable bowel, cancer, chronic viral infections, ear infections, chronic fatigue

- Larch arabinogalactan (LA) is a polysaccharide and a source of dietary fibre in the form of a fine white powder extracted from the wood, particularly Western Larch. Recent studies have shown it to be anti-inflammatory, effective in stimulating the immune system and increasing the body's ability to defend itself against viral infections. LA may increase levels of beneficial intestinal anaerobes, macrophages, and T-cells, stimulate Natural Killer Cell cytotoxicity, and increase release of interferon, holding promise in treatment of many diseases, such as Alzheimer's, irritable bowel syndrome, ear infections, chronic fatigue, and the common cold.
- Traditional uses of the bark and needles were in decoctions for sore throat, inflamed gums, coughs, colds, and digestive disorders, or as a wash for wounds, rashes, psoriasis, or eczema. Spring needles are rich in Vitamin C. Resin is applied to the skin for cuts and bruises or chewed for sore throats.

OTHER USES:
- Gum is a thickening agent.
- Sap can be boiled down to make a syrup.
- The bark contains tannins.
- Wood is used for building material, as it doesn't rot as fast as other wood.

INFUSION: Gather fresh spring tips, cover with boiling water, and steep, covered, for 20 minutes. Drink as desired.

LEMON BALM

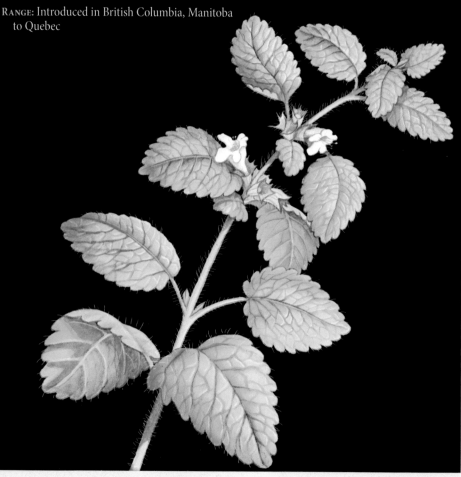

Melissa officinalis

FAMILY: Lamiaceae

OTHER NAMES: Sweet Balm, *Fr.* Mélisse

PARTS USED: Leaves

CHARACTERISTICS: Sour, spicy, cool

SYSTEMS AFFECTED: Lungs, liver

ACTIONS: Diaphoretic, antimicrobial, antispasmodic, carminative, emmenagogue, stomachic, febrifuge, nervine, sedative

RANGE: Introduced in British Columbia, Manitoba to Quebec

A native of southern Europe, this perennial now grows all over the world, although here it is mostly found in gardens or old homesteads rather than in the wild. The name Melissa stems from the Greek word for honey, and was probably used because of bees' attraction to it. It grows from 30–60 cm. high and has fine hairs; the leaves are opposite, oval, and wrinkled with scalloped edges, and when rubbed give off a lemony scent. The stem is square and branched, the flowers appear in small bunches around the leaf axils and bloom from June to October. The plant dies down in winter but the root is perennial. Harvest in the afternoon in early summer when the oils are strongest. Best if tinctured fresh.

MEDICINAL USES:
Stress, insomnia, indigestion, wounds, cold sores

- Has a tonic effect on the heart, slightly lowering blood pressure and easing tension, depression, anxiety, palpitations. Research in clinical studies shows that Lemon Balm is effective in helping promote sleep, particularly when added to other sleep-inducing herbs. Relieves muscle spasms, increases calmness and alertness, and improves memory.
- Soothes upset stomach, especially where there is anxiety; relieves gas; and promotes appetite. Drink a tea before meals to help digestion. Taking a mixture of Lemon Balm, Fennel, and Chamomile before breastfeeding helps to calm a colicky baby.
- Used by Indigenous Peoples in preparations for colds, fever, and chills; induces perspiration.
- Used in ointments to prevent and relieve cold sores and herpes lesions, ulcers, to heal open wounds, stop bleeding.
- Leaves steeped in wine were once used to relieve insect bites and stings.

OTHER USES:
- Can be used in pesto, or as a flavouring for soups, beverages, or salads.
- Makes an effective bug spray.

INFUSION: 1 tsp. dried herb in 1 cup of boiling water. Drink up to 4 times a day. For insomnia, add valerian. For cold sores, steep 2–4 tsp. crushed herb in 1 cup boiling water. Cool and apply with cotton swabs throughout the day.

TINCTURE: 60 drops daily.

CALMING TEA:

4 parts Lemon Balm

3 parts Chamomile

2 parts Skullcap

1 part Motherwort

Use 2–3 tsp. to 1 cup boiling water. Steep for 10 minutes.

CAUTION: May interact with sedatives and thyroid medications, or if you are taking drugs for HIV. Not recommended during pregnancy. Consult your doctor if you are taking any medications.

LOBELIA

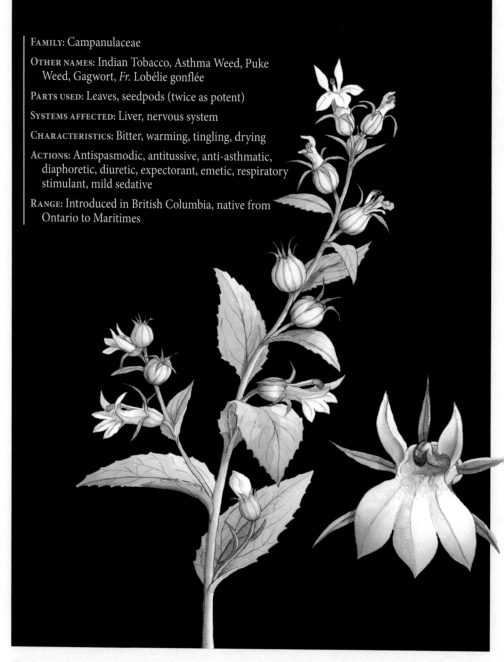

Lobelia inflata

FAMILY: Campanulaceae

OTHER NAMES: Indian Tobacco, Asthma Weed, Puke Weed, Gagwort, *Fr.* Lobélie gonflée

PARTS USED: Leaves, seedpods (twice as potent)

SYSTEMS AFFECTED: Liver, nervous system

CHARACTERISTICS: Bitter, warming, tingling, drying

ACTIONS: Antispasmodic, antitussive, anti-asthmatic, diaphoretic, diuretic, expectorant, emetic, respiratory stimulant, mild sedative

RANGE: Introduced in British Columbia, native from Ontario to Maritimes

This controversial herb is often known by the names Pukeweed or Gagwort, giving us a clue to its powerful emetic properties. However, its real talent lies in its use as an antispasmodic, particularly in cases of asthma or dry, spasmodic coughs. One of the most disputed herbs in the world, it is either feared as being highly toxic and even deadly, or regarded as a miracle herb that can cure even the most hopeless cases. Its use began with Indigenous Peoples of North America, but its popularity in western herbalism started in the 1800s with Samuel Thomson, who claimed it was a "diffusive" which could clear blockages in the life force, arousing or sedating, depending on what was needed. It has a tendency to enhance the effects of other medicines when used in small amounts in compounds, directing them to where they need to go. This is a herb that should not be used by anyone unless they are experienced in its correct and safe use.

An erect annual/biennial that grows 30–60 cm. high, its slightly hairy stem is simple or branched with delicate lavender, pale blue, or white tubular flowers in terminal clusters. Its leaves are alternate, toothed, and lance-shaped. The fruit forms inside a globular "inflated" capsule that splits open when ripe. They should be harvested after these pods have appeared but before they split, and dried for later use. It loses its potency rather quickly once dried. Store out of sunlight.

MEDICINAL USES:

Asthma, dry spasmodic coughs, bronchitis, food poisoning, stings, body aches, stiff neck

- Powerful antispasmodic, dilates bronchial passages easing asthma and bronchitis, dry coughs, pneumonia.
- Diffusive relaxant, it can equalize the circulation of blood, reaching almost every tissue in the body and influencing the nerves and muscles, relieving all types of pain due to muscle spasm. Mild sedative, it slows respiration and lowers blood pressure.
- Potent emetic, it will induce vomiting if used in too large a dose.
- Once used to quit smoking, it contains lobeline, a nicotine-like substance that is not addictive; however if used along with tobacco products, Lobelia's toxic effects may be enhanced so it is not recommended.
- When used externally, the leaves can be applied as a poultice to ease the pain of stings, bites, body aches, and stiff neck.

ACID TINCTURE: Add 4 tbsp. crushed seed and 4 tbsp. dried herb powder to 2 cups malt vinegar or apple cider vinegar. (To increase efficacy, add ½ tsp. Cayenne powder to stimulate or ground Ginger root to relax). Cover and macerate for 10–14 days, shaking periodically. Filter out herbal matter, add 2 tbsp. alcohol, bottle, and label. Start with 1–3 drops, and titrate up from there for next dose, stopping when desired effect is achieved or if nausea occurs. Do not exceed 10 drops per day.

COMBINATIONS:

A few drops of Acid Tincture may be added to Horehound, Hyssop, or Sage teas for asthma and coughs. Works well with Skullcap, Black Cohosh, and/or Skunk Cabbage for spasms or cramps.

CAUTION: Toxic in large doses. May cause vomiting, sweating, diarrhea, tremors, rapid heartbeat, mental confusion, convulsions. Avoid in pregnancy, high blood pressure, heart, liver or kidney disease. May cause irritation in the digestive tract. Use only under supervision of a professional.

MULLEIN

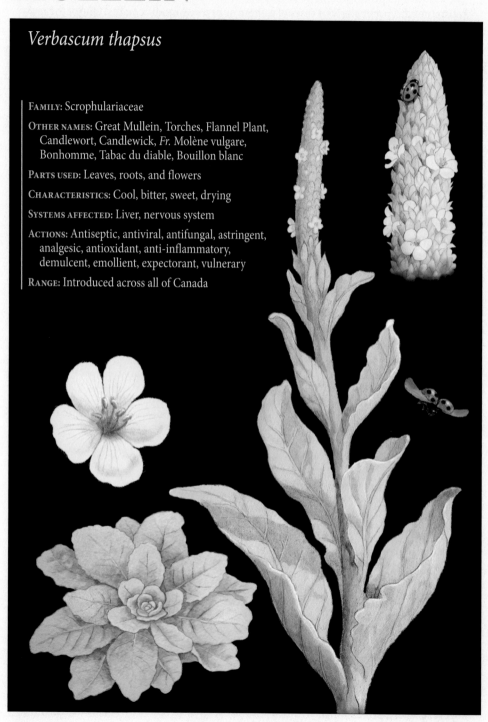

Verbascum thapsus

FAMILY: Scrophulariaceae

OTHER NAMES: Great Mullein, Torches, Flannel Plant, Candlewort, Candlewick, *Fr.* Molène vulgare, Bonhomme, Tabac du diable, Bouillon blanc

PARTS USED: Leaves, roots, and flowers

CHARACTERISTICS: Cool, bitter, sweet, drying

SYSTEMS AFFECTED: Liver, nervous system

ACTIONS: Antiseptic, antiviral, antifungal, astringent, analgesic, antioxidant, anti-inflammatory, demulcent, emollient, expectorant, vulnerary

RANGE: Introduced across all of Canada

Mullein is a hard plant to miss as it often grows to a height of 1.5–1.8 metres. During the first season of growth, only a rosette of soft, hairy leaves up to 38 cm. long appears, then the following spring a hairy stalk emerges from the centre, with leaves joined to the stalk becoming smaller towards the top. The top becomes a flower spike, usually about a foot long, with flowers blooming randomly along the stalk. The flowers are composed of 5 petals, about 2.5 cm. in diameter. They should be harvested and dried quickly and carefully so as not to bruise the delicate petals, since this will diminish their efficacy. Take only a few leaves so as not to kill the plant.

MEDICINAL USES:

Chest colds, bronchitis, asthma, earaches, and eczema

- Ideal for reducing inflammation in the respiratory tract. It may tone the mucous membranes, stimulate fluid production, and relax the gut wall to make expectoration easier. This works well in bronchitis where there is a hard, dry cough with soreness. Also works for chest colds, asthma, and laryngitis.
- Fresh leaves work externally as a poultice to ease pain, bruising, itching, and to heal slow-healing wounds, burns, rashes, tumours and hemorrhoids. Also used topically to ease pain from arthritis, swelling, or broken bones.
- Oil made by macerating flowers in olive oil is quite effective in relieving earache or eczema in the ear as well as in treating gum and mouth ulcers. It also works on the scalp to keep it free from dandruff and to condition hair.
- Some Indigenous Peoples smoke the leaves to treat asthma, or steep them in water and inhale the vapours.
- An extract from the roots can relieve toothache pain.

OTHER USES:
- Used in cosmetics to soften the skin.
- The leaves were once stuffed in shoes to keep feet warm.
- A yellow dye can be made from the flowers.
- Also used as a hair rinse.

FOLKLORE: The stem stripped of leaves and dipped in tallow was used as a torch and to protect against enchantment. Smoked leaves were believed to clear the air of negative energies and often used in witches' ceremonies. The leaves were even carried to prevent conception.

INFUSION FOR COUGHS: One ounce of dried leaves may be boiled for 10 minutes in a pint of milk and strained thoroughly to remove the tiny hairs and plant material. This is given warm with honey to relieve cough. May be combined with Coltsfoot and/or Thyme.

TINCTURE: Standard, 1–2 ml. every few hours as needed.

EAR OIL: For earaches, or eczema in the ear. Cut blooms into small pieces, place in a small glass jar, cover with organic extra virgin olive oil. Mix well and mash with wooden spoon. Add a few drops of vitamin E oil. Cover and shake. Put in a dark place and macerate for 6 weeks, shaking often. Strain well and pour into dark coloured jar. Store at room temperature. To use, place 2–3 drops in ear 2–3 times a day.

CAUTION: Preparations using leaves and taken internally should be strained through a fine cloth or sieve to remove tiny hairs which can be irritant to the digestive tract. Not recommended during pregnancy or if taking anti-diabetic or diuretic medications.

OLD MAN'S BEARD

Usnea barbata
U. longissima

FAMILY: Parmeliaceae

OTHER NAMES: Usnea, Beard Lichen, Witch's Hair, *Fr.* Usnée barbue

PARTS USED: Whole lichen

CHARACTERISTICS: Bitter, dry, cool

ACTIONS: Antibacterial, antiviral, antifungal, astringent, styptic, tonic, vulnerary

RANGE: *U. barbata* native across all of Canada; *U. longissima* native to British Columbia, Ontario to Newfoundland

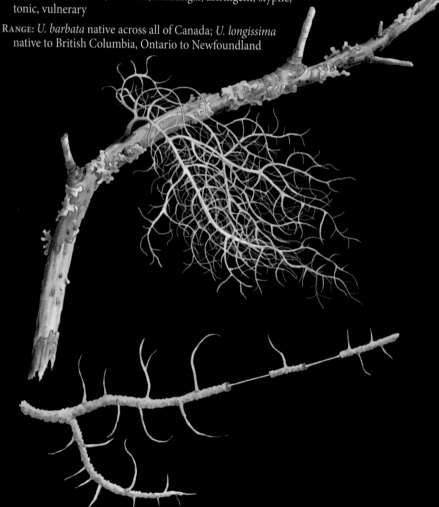

Usnea, or Old Man's Beard, is a greenish-grey lichen, an organism that has a symbiotic relationship between algae and fungi. It grows on the branches of older trees, often ones that are sick or dying, and can be distinguished from other similar-looking lichens by a white elastic thread (fungus) running through the middle that is revealed by gently pulling apart a filament (algae). There are hundreds of species, and it has been used for centuries worldwide as a powerful antimicrobial—that is, it is effective against a wide range of pathogens. *U. barbata* can grow up to 20 cm. long, *U. longissima* much longer, and since it is very slow growing it should be harvested from dead or fallen branches to avoid over-harvesting. Choose a clean location as it easily absorbs heavy metals and pollution from the environment. Store in a dry place; chop finely before using.

MEDICINAL USES:
Bacterial, viral, and fungal infections, wounds

- Used on a wide range of diseases, and as it can kill pathogens without disrupting most gut flora, it is a valuable prevention and treatment for many infections, both viral and bacterial. Effective against gram-positive bacteria like Streptococcus and Staphylococcus, as well as pneumonia, upper respiratory tract infections, and urinary tract infections, but unlike most antibiotics, it won't kill off healthy gut bacteria. Combats common viral infections such as herpes and Epstein–Barr. It works through the mucous membranes to fight lung and bronchial infections that cause yellow or green phlegm and fevers.
- Effective, both topically and internally, against fungal infections like candida, athlete's foot, and ringworm, although lifestyle and diet modifications should be made in order to completely eradicate such infections, as they are usually hard to get rid of.
- May be useful in treatment for gastric ulcers and shows potential as a possible cancer treatment.
- Used topically on wounds to heal and prevent infection.

FOLKLORE: Seen by many Indigenous peoples of North America as having a sacred relationship with the trees, helping them fight off infection.

TINCTURE (DUAL EXTRACTION): Place ¼ cup chopped fresh or dried herb into a pot with ½ cup water. Bring to a boil, cover and simmer 15–20 minutes until reduced to ⅓ cup. Cool for a few minutes and pour into a Mason jar. Add ⅓ cup 70% alcohol and mix well. Screw on lid and let sit for 2 weeks, shaking daily to mix. Strain and transfer to amber tincture bottle. Take 6–12 drops 3 times a day.

CAUTION: Avoid during pregnancy. May irritate the digestive system in large amounts.

OREGON GRAPE

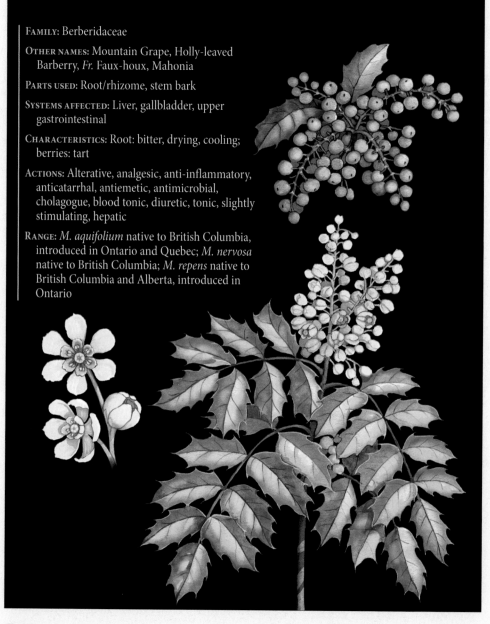

Mahonia aquifolium
M. nervosa (Cascade)
M. repens (Creeping)

FAMILY: Berberidaceae

OTHER NAMES: Mountain Grape, Holly-leaved Barberry, *Fr.* Faux-houx, Mahonia

PARTS USED: Root/rhizome, stem bark

SYSTEMS AFFECTED: Liver, gallbladder, upper gastrointestinal

CHARACTERISTICS: Root: bitter, drying, cooling; berries: tart

ACTIONS: Alterative, analgesic, anti-inflammatory, anticatarrhal, antiemetic, antimicrobial, cholagogue, blood tonic, diuretic, tonic, slightly stimulating, hepatic

RANGE: *M. aquifolium* native to British Columbia, introduced in Ontario and Quebec; *M. nervosa* native to British Columbia; *M. repens* native to British Columbia and Alberta, introduced in Ontario

A n ornamental evergreen shrub that typically grows in mountainous country of up to 2,000 metres, Oregon Grape belongs to the Barberry family, known for its bitter alkaloid berberine. Growing 2–3 metres tall, it has shiny leaves that look similar to Holly; however, they are pinnately arranged, with 5–11 ovate leaflets. Dark green on top and lighter underneath, they have spiny tips on the toothed edges and turn reddish in the fall. The yellow, scented flowers bloom in early spring in terminal clusters, then in summer the dark blue berries appear, covered in a dusty coating. They are quite tart but edible and make a nice jelly or jam when sugar is added. The bark of stems, roots, and rhizomes is bright yellow when you scrape off the surface, and should be collected in late fall or early spring, paying special attention to not kill the plant by taking only a small part of the root or stem. Chop up while fresh and dry for future use.

MEDICINAL USES:

Digestive weakness, lack of appetite, skin diseases, bacterial dysentery, infected wounds, syphilis

- Contains an alkaloid called berberine which tends to cool, drain, and detoxify, improving inflammatory and stagnant conditions. Some studies are showing Oregon Grape root can actually decrease bacterial resistance to antibiotics and increase antibiotic effectiveness.
- A bitter liver and gallbladder tonic, it stimulates the digestion and bile flow, improving liver function and purifying the blood of toxins. This action also helps loss of appetite, gastritis, digestive weakness, IBS, and diarrhea, and improves absorption of nutrients. Root is antibacterial and can treat enteric infections like bacterial dysentery.
- Noted for its effectiveness for treating skin diseases such as psoriasis, eczema, acne, and dermatitis when added to creams or salves.
- Fruit is a gentle laxative.
- Infusion may be used as a gargle for sore throats.
- Indicated for any abnormal discharges, phlegm, catarrh, leukorrhea or candida where there is heat and inflammation.

OTHER USES:
- Yellow dye made from bark and roots, dark green and purple dyes from the fruit.
- Berries are tart but can be made into jams or jellies.

TINCTURE: 1 part roots and bark dried and ground to 5 parts alcohol, macerate up to 30 days, drain, and bottle. Take 10–60 drops 3 times a day.

COMBINATIONS:

Cascara Sagrada for chronic constipation, Pipsissewa for hepatitis, jaundice and arthritis. Licorice root should not be used in combinations as it nullifies the effects of Oregon Grape root.

CAUTION: Avoid use for more than 2 weeks, not recommended for children, pregnant or lactating women. Avoid in hyperthyroidism. High doses may cause vomiting, low blood pressure, reduced heart rate, lethargy, skin and eye irritation, kidney infection.

PACIFIC HEMLOCK

Tsuga heterophylla
T. mertensiana (Mountain Hemlock)

FAMILY: Pinaceae

OTHER NAMES: Western Hemlock, *Fr.* Pruche de l'Ouest, Tsuga de l'Ouest

PARTS USED: Light green tips, inner bark, resin

SYSTEMS AFFECTED: Urinary

CHARACTERISTICS: Sweet, pungent

ACTIONS: Antioxidant, antimicrobial, astringent, diuretic, diaphoretic

RANGE: *T. heterophylla* native to British Columbia and Alberta;
T. mertensiana native to British Columbia

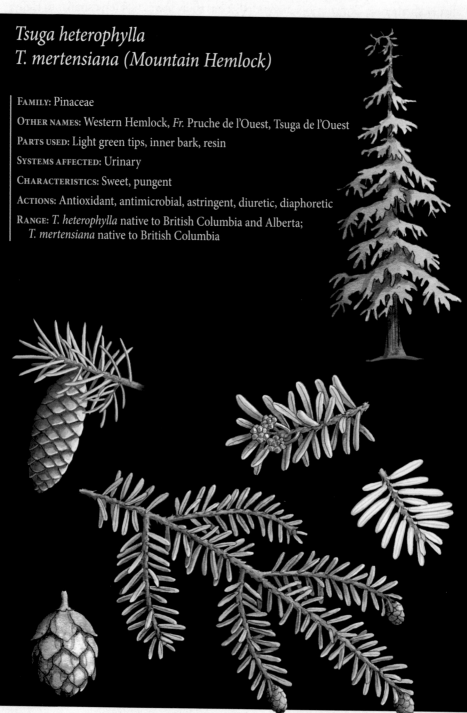

This native conifer has been long considered an important female medicine by the Coast Salish of British Columbia. Although the name brings to mind the poisonous herb (Conium maculatum) that killed Socrates, it is in no way poisonous, and it was simply given the name because of its odour, which resembles that of the herb. One of the tallest and most common evergreens in Western BC and Alaska, it has been known to grow up to 83 metres, although it usually ranges around 60 metres, its trunk measuring up to 2.7 metres in diameter. It's usually recognizable by its drooping, feathery crown, as well as the blunt needles of varying lengths with two white stripes on their underside. The male cones are tiny and yellow, the female cones are 2–5 cm. in length and can be purple-green when young or brown as they get older. The bark also changes with age, being reddish brown and smooth when young and becoming grey and more furrowed as it ages. It is tolerant of a wide variety of growing conditions, and has been known to reach 1,200 years of age. Collect bark only from branches that are close to the ground and within reach so as not to harm the tree. Light green branch tips can be harvested in the spring and used fresh.

MEDICINAL USES:

Hemorrhages, tuberculosis, kidney and bladder problems, diarrhea, colds, fever

- Bark can be peeled easily from young branches; inner bark is scraped off, pounded, and dried to be used as medicine or food.
- Infusion or decoction of the inner bark or twigs is diuretic and astringent, used internally for kidney and bladder complaints, diarrhea, hemorrhaging, tuberculosis, and fevers.
- Used externally in a decoction of the bark for sores, ulcers, or rashes, or in a poultice for bleeding wounds. Indigenous Peoples including the Nuxalk also chew the needles and use them as a poultice for burns.
- Sap or resin can be heated with fat to make a salve or with oil as a chest rub for colds and sore muscles. Some Indigenous people, specifically the Nuxalk, apply warm sap to wounds or use it in a poultice to ease the pain of rheumatism.
- Needles are rich in Vitamin C and can be drunk as an infusion.

OTHER USES:
- Inner bark dried to a powder and used as thickener for soups or mixed with flours for bread.
- Pounded and steamed into a paste, it is used to make cakes, often mixed with berries and roasted in a pit oven or eaten in winter as survival food.
- Powdered bark is put into shoes for sweaty feet and to reduce foot odour.
- Wood is often carved for utensils. The bark is rich in tannin and used for tanning hides, and it also yields a red or brown dye.
- Macerate the tips in sugar, then use the sugar in baked goods or for deglazing roasted meat.

BARK DECOCTION: Drink ½–¾ cups up to 3 times a day.

TIP INFUSION: Standard infusion, drink ½–¾ cups up to 3 times a day.

OIL: Place 2 tbsp. ground pitch into a Mason jar with 1 cup of olive oil; a few twigs may be added if desired. Place in a crockpot with a couple of inches of water and heat for 3 or 4 days at 100–120°F, strain and bottle.

PACIFIC MADRONE

Arbutus menziesii

FAMILY: Ericaceae

OTHER NAMES: Madrona, Pacific Arbutus, *Fr.* Arbousier d'Amérique

PARTS USED: Leaves, bark

SYSTEMS AFFECTED: Urinary

CHARACTERISTICS: Spicy, pungent

ACTIONS: Stomachic, vulnerary, astringent

RANGE: Native to southern British Columbia coastline

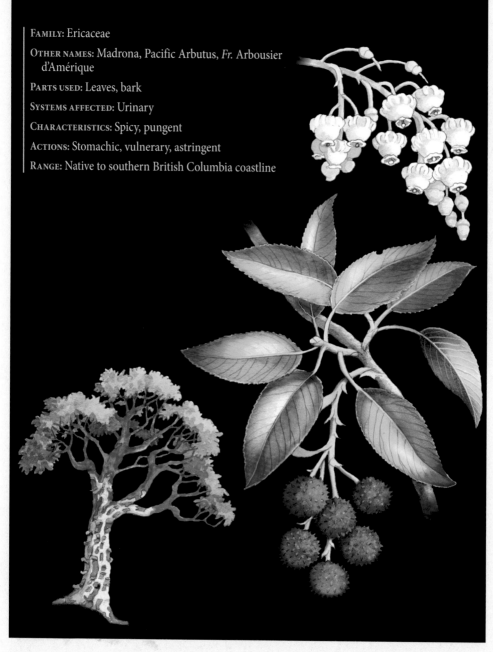

The Pacific Madrone or Arbutus is found growing near sea level in the extreme south-west of British Columbia. Preferring dry, open, well-drained forests along the coastline, it is the only broad-leaved evergreen tree in Canada. Easily recognizable by its thin, papery, reddish-brown bark that peels off in curls and strips exposing its smooth green or silvery wood underneath, it can grow up to 30 metres tall, although typically shorter. It is known to rely on forest fires to open up the understorey, reducing competition so it can re-sprout from an underground burl, even after being destroyed aboveground. Its thick, glossy leaves are alternate and oval-shaped, with finely toothed or smooth edges, and turn from dark green to red-orange in the second year, falling off once the second year's growth has appeared. Its fragrant, urn-shaped flowers bloom from April to May and are designed to attract bees, growing in terminal drooping clusters. The red berry that appears later in the summer and into the fall has a bumpy surface with hooked barbs that cling to passersby. Its astringent and mealy taste is not usually found palatable by humans, although wildlife love them, and they are sometimes used to make cider or jellies. Harvest leaf clusters from branch tips from mid-spring to fall; berries should be fully red before picking. Dry and store for future use.

MEDICINAL USES:

Bladder infections, stomachache, sore throat, skin inflammations, vaginal yeast infections

- Bark and leaves contain tannins that make an astringent decoction useful in treating bladder infections, stomachaches, cramps, colds, and sore throats. Leaves may be chewed for the same ailments.
- An infusion of the bark can be used for skin ailments such as impetigo, sores, burns, and cuts. Reduces redness and leaves skin soft and smooth, closing the pores. Fresh crushed leaves can be applied directly to burns or sores. A cup of infusion can be added to a sitz bath for vaginal inflammation and yeast infections.

OTHER USES:
- Tannins in bark used as a preservative for wood and ropes, tanning leather, and as a source of brown dye.
- Bark dried and ground to use as a spice, having a taste somewhere between cinnamon and mushrooms with a hint of fruitiness.
- Dried berries can be ground into powder as a spice or sugar substitute, or strung into necklaces.

TINCTURE: 1 part dried leaf to 5 parts vodka, macerate for 1 month, drain, and bottle. Take 30–60 drops in 1 cup water, up to 3 times a day.

CAUTION: Not for use during pregnancy. Restrict internal use to 4–6 days.

PACIFIC YEW

Taxus brevifolia

FAMILY: Taxaceae

OTHER NAMES: Western Yew, *Fr.* If de l'Ouest, If Occidental

PARTS USED: Bark, leaves

ACTIONS: Anticancer, diaphoretic

RANGE: Native to British Columbia and Southwestern Alberta

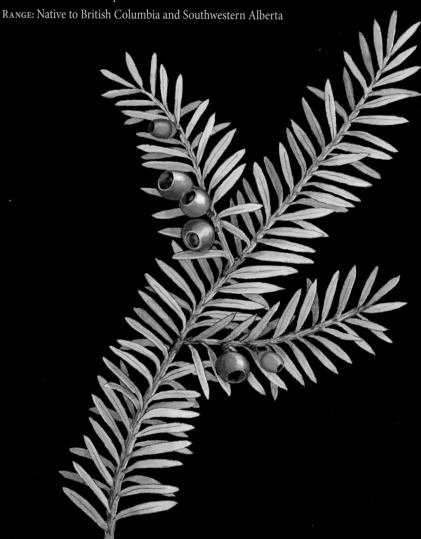

Thought to be one of the oldest trees on earth, the Yew was once considered a symbol of death and eternal life in the British Isles, and was held sacred by the Druids, who often built their temples beside them. The Pacific Yew is an evergreen shrub or small tree that grows in the damp forests of the Pacific Northwest. Although it was once used medicinally by Indigenous Peoples in North America for various ailments, it was never used in western herbalism as the entire plant is poisonous, including the hard seed of the red berry but excluding the fleshy part surrounding it. In the 1960s, the National Cancer Institute began testing the bark as a possible cure for cancer and found that it contained a compound called paclitaxel, which can inhibit mitosis or cell division in cancer cells. It was found to effectively treat patients with breast, ovarian, and lung cancers and is now marketed as Taxol, used for a variety of cancer types. Since Pacific Yew is such a slow-growing tree and it requires several full-grown trees to extract enough for one patient, supply and demand is a problem. It has been harvested almost to extinction in North America, but with new research into alternate species, creating synthetic or semi-synthetic substitutes, and using endophytic fungus as an alternate source, some of the pressure has been taken off a fragile population.

MEDICINAL USES:

Cancer, rheumatism, amenorrhea

- Traditionally used by Indigenous Peoples for poultices on wounds and rheumatism, or as a tea for menstrual cramps, fever, and stomachaches. However, any form of internal use is strongly discouraged due to its high toxicity.
- Use as a cancer drug is very effective, although there are several side effects, such as hair loss, nausea, vomiting, and joint and muscle pain. It can only be used under supervision of a qualified healthcare professional.

OTHER USES: Durable wood, used by Indigenous Peoples for making tools that are likely to endure a lot of stress, such as paddles, bows, harpoons, sewing needles, knives, and snowshoes.

CAUTION: All parts of the plant are extremely toxic, except for the red flesh of the berry. Ingestion of only 50–100 grams of needles can be fatal. Not suitable for self-medication.

PIPSISSEWA

Chimaphila umbellata

FAMILY: Ericaceae

OTHER NAMES: Prince's Pine, Winter Green, Butter Winter, Ground Holly, *Fr.* Chimaphile à ombelles, Herbe à clef, Pyrole en ombelle

PARTS USED: Leaves

SYSTEMS AFFECTED: Kidneys, lymph

CHARACTERISTICS: Sweet, slightly bitter, warming

ACTIONS: Alterative, antibacterial, antioxidant, antifungal, astringent, diuretic, diaphoretic, rubefacient, stimulant, tonic

RANGE: Native across all of Canada, except Nunavut and Labrador

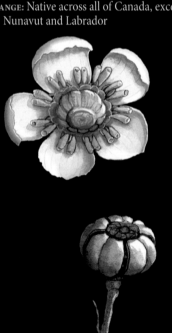

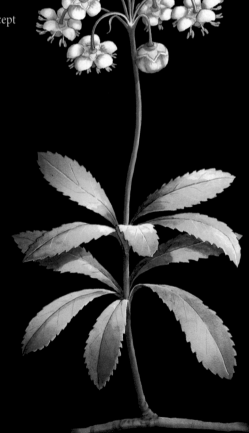

This small native perennial evergreen is found growing in well-drained coniferous forests and woodlands of low to middle elevations throughout Canada. Shade-tolerant and in need of a specific mycorrhizal association in order to thrive, it is not easy to grow and has become rare in certain parts of the country due to overharvesting. The name Pipsissewa comes from the Cree word meaning "break into small pieces," referring to its ability to break up kidney stones. It grows to a height of 10–25 cm., and has creeping yellow rhizomes with several erect stems and shiny, dark-green toothed leaves that appear to grow in whorls around it. The five-petalled pink or purplish flowers are waxy and fragrant, appearing from July to August, and the fruit, an erect dark-brown capsule with five sections, remains, eventually cracking open to disperse its seeds. The upper leaves may be harvested before flowering, but be careful not to over-harvest. Leave the roots intact and avoid trampling the surrounding soil. Dry carefully, preferably in a dehydrator, in order to retain the green colour and its medicinal properties.

MEDICINAL USES:
Bladder and kidney disorders, rheumatism, gout

- Contains hydroquinone, which helps disinfect the urinary tract and ease the symptoms of cystitis and urethritis and break up bladder or kidney stones. Strengthens the bladder and helps with incontinence and bedwetting.
- Diuretic; used in infusion or decoction it removes inflammatory toxins from the body, helping with arthritis, rheumatism, and gout.
- Stimulates the removal of waste through the lymphatic system, helps swollen glands and hardened, inflamed lymph nodes, relieves stagnation.
- Used by some Indigenous Peoples for colds, coughs, fevers, arthritis, bladder infections, stones, stomach aches, rheumatism, and back pain.
- Decoction or compresses or warm, fresh leaves can be applied topically to relieve pain from arthritis.

OTHER USES: Flavouring for candies, soft drinks.

TINCTURE: Fresh 1:2, dried 1:5, in 50% alcohol. Take 20–40 drops up to 4 times a day. For kidney stones, take 5–10 drops every 3 hours.

INFUSION: Standard, ½–1 cup 2–3 times a day.

COMBINATIONS:

Some Indigenous Peoples combined Pipsissewa with Mullein to relieve bedwetting in children. Use with Agrimony and Corn Silk for bladder infections. Combine with False Unicorn Root and Partridge Berry for leukorrhea.

CAUTION: Avoid long-term use. Fresh leaves may cause irritation or blistering in some people.

PLANTAIN

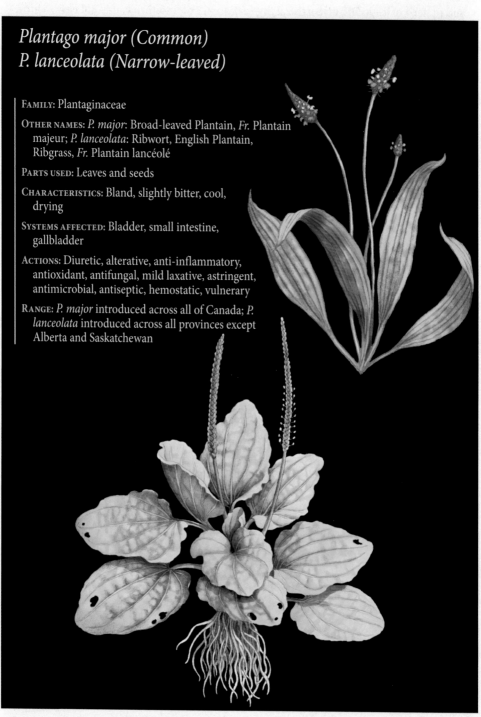

Plantago major (Common)
P. lanceolata (Narrow-leaved)

FAMILY: Plantaginaceae

OTHER NAMES: *P. major*: Broad-leaved Plantain, *Fr.* Plantain majeur; *P. lanceolata*: Ribwort, English Plantain, Ribgrass, *Fr.* Plantain lancéolé

PARTS USED: Leaves and seeds

CHARACTERISTICS: Bland, slightly bitter, cool, drying

SYSTEMS AFFECTED: Bladder, small intestine, gallbladder

ACTIONS: Diuretic, alterative, anti-inflammatory, antioxidant, antifungal, mild laxative, astringent, antimicrobial, antiseptic, hemostatic, vulnerary

RANGE: *P. major* introduced across all of Canada; *P. lanceolata* introduced across all provinces except Alberta and Saskatchewan

One of our most common herbs found in Canada, Plantain is seen growing on practically every lawn, roadside, or abandoned lot. Originally from Europe, it was traditionally used on the battlefield to staunch wounds. It will grow virtually anywhere, including paved driveways or in sidewalk cracks, and needs very little sun. It grows close to the ground, with a rosette of ovate, blunt leaves 10–25 cm. long, with long, fibrous ribs. The erect flower spikes are dark green and can be up to 30 cm. long. The Narrow-leaved Plantain (*P. lanceolata*) has narrower leaves and longer-stemmed flower spikes but has much the same medicinal properties as the common variety. The young plants may be eaten in salads in the spring; to preserve for later they should be gathered during flowering throughout the summer and dried quickly as they will tend to discolour rapidly. Use only plants from yards that have never been sprayed with chemicals.

MEDICINAL USES:

Wounds, insect bites, urinary tract infections, digestive tract inflammations

- Bruised leaves may be applied directly to stings or insect bites, sunburn, or acne, or used in a salve or ointment; soothes and relieves pain and itching.
- Astringent, stops bleeding, promotes healing of exterior wounds; rich in tannin, which helps draw tissues together.
- Heals urinary tract infections and other internal inflammations including hepatitis.
- Tea brewed from leaves and the seeds, which are high in mucilage, is a folk remedy for colitis, diarrhea, dysentery, and bleeding hemorrhoids. It is also antispasmodic, reducing cramping. Seeds also act as a laxative, its mucilage repairing irritated intestinal membranes.
- Infusion of the leaves and seeds also used as a gentle expectorant, to soothe an inflamed throat, or to ease gastric inflammation, ulcers, and bleeding mucous membranes.
- Studies indicate that Plantain may also reduce blood pressure and lower cholesterol.
- Leaves are high in calcium and vitamins A, C, and K. Combines well with Calendula, Yarrow, Chamomile, and Agrimony in infusions for healing.
- Leaves may be heated in warm water and applied to swollen joints or sore muscles.

OTHER USES:
- Cold tea used as a hair rinse for dandruff.
- Once believed to cure rabies and ward off snakes.
- Put on aching feet after a long trek to relieve soreness and fatigue.

HEALING SALVE: Place ½ pound of entire chopped Plantain plant in a non-metallic pan, add ½ cup lard or coconut oil, heat slowly on low heat until it becomes green and wilted, strain, pour into jars, and cool. For use on burns, rashes, bites, and other sores.

COMBINATIONS:

Root combined with White Horehound used traditionally for rattlesnake bites. Works well with Comfrey and Calendula in a healing salve.

PONDEROSA PINE

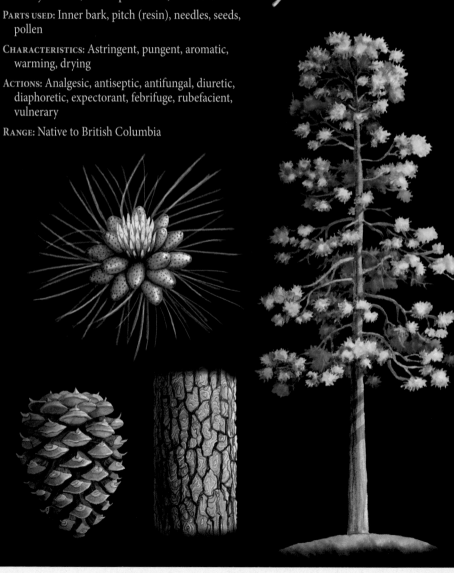

Pinus ponderosa

FAMILY: Pinaceae

OTHER NAMES: Western Yellow Pine, Washoe Pine, Blackjack Pine, *Fr.* Pin ponderosa, Pin lourd

PARTS USED: Inner bark, pitch (resin), needles, seeds, pollen

CHARACTERISTICS: Astringent, pungent, aromatic, warming, drying

ACTIONS: Analgesic, antiseptic, antifungal, diuretic, diaphoretic, expectorant, febrifuge, rubefacient, vulnerary

RANGE: Native to British Columbia

This majestic, fragrant evergreen is revered by the western Indigenous communities for its medicinal properties and its usefulness as building material. The name Ponderosa means "heavy or large" in Latin. With its straight trunk it towers over other trees to a height of 30–40 metres or more and can live up to six hundred years, its base reaching 1–2 metres in diameter. It is distinguished from other pines by its long, toothed, yellowish-green needles (12–28 cm.) in bundles of three, and its brown or cinnamon-coloured bark that breaks apart easily in pieces resembling a jigsaw puzzle, the dark fissures growing deeper as it ages. Its thick bark makes it particularly resistant to low-intensity forest fires. The cones are egg-shaped with a sharp spike pointing outward at the tip of each scale and contain the seeds, or pine nuts, which are eaten as food. It prefers well-drained soil and is shade intolerant. Its roots extend deep into the earth in search of water. The best time to harvest is in the spring, using the young needles for tea and taking a low-hanging branch for its inner bark, being careful not to strip more than a few square inches off the main trunk, as it can kill the tree. The yellow pollen is harvested from the male cones in the spring; harvest them slightly before they open, then bring them inside to dry in a warm space. They will open and release the pollen. Store in a bottle in the freezer to preserve freshness.

MEDICINAL USES:

Lung or sinus congestion and coughs, joint and muscle pain, fevers, sores or cuts, low energy and immunity

- Infusion of needles, inner bark, and/or pitch is rich in Vitamin A and C, opens up sinuses, breaks up green, sticky phlegm, increasing secretions to help coughs.
- Pitch, when slightly warmed to soften, can be chewed for sore throats, coughs.
- Pitch can be used in ointments or salves for sores, boils, or cuts, or to draw out splinters. It will also ease the pain of rheumatism or sore back.
- A decoction of the young branch tips is used for internal bleeding and high fevers.
- Infusion of dried buds can be used as an eyewash.
- Pollen contains phytoandrogens, which are hormones that mimic the ones naturally occurring in our bodies. They can increase stamina, help with the aging process, decrease inflammation, and improve immunity. Consider as a steroid, and cycle usage on and off to avoid side effects like acne.

OTHER USES:
- Wood used for construction, building canoes, and in sweat lodges.
- Pitch used to waterproof and preserve wood.
- Seeds and inner bark can be dried and ground to add to soups and breads.

TINCTURE: Resin, 1:2, in 95% alcohol. Take 20–60 drops up to 4 times a day. Add honey if desired.

OIL: 1 part resin to 5 parts oil (olive, grapeseed, or almond). Let sit in a warm place for 3 weeks. For salve, add 28 grams of beeswax to warmed infused oil, adjust to desired consistency.

INFUSION: Needles: standard, 4–8 tbsp. up to 3 times a day. Bark or pitch may be added to increase effectiveness.

CAUTION: Avoid using resins if you have kidney problems. Avoid during pregnancy.

QUEEN ANNE'S LACE

Daucus carota

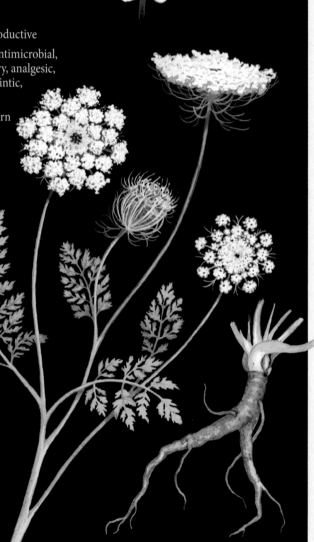

FAMILY: Apiaceae

OTHER NAMES: Wild Carrot, Bee's Nest, Bird's Nest, *Fr.* Carotte sauvage

PARTS USED: Root, leaves, and seeds

CHARACTERISTICS: Bitter

SYSTEMS AFFECTED: Urinary, reproductive

ACTIONS: Diuretic, antioxidant, antimicrobial, hypotensive, anti-inflammatory, analgesic, purgative, vermifuge, anthelmintic, carminative, antilithic

RANGE: Introduced across southern provinces.

This biennial herb found along roadsides and fields throughout most of southern Canada during the summer months is a direct descendant of our garden carrot. A native of southern Europe, its stems are up to 90 cm. high, erect and branched, with finely dissected, fern-like leaves. Flowers are densely clustered white umbels radiating from the central stalk with a tiny purple or pink flower in the centre. As the seeds ripen, the umbels contract and curve inwards, forming a nest-like appearance, hence the name Bird's Nest. The large taproot is whitish and bitter and smells like carrot. It is harvested in late summer and should be cut longitudinally and dried or the tender smaller roots may be eaten fresh in the spring. The leaves should be picked in July before it has gone to seed, as the seeds are more potent when collected just before they are fully mature.

MEDICINAL USES:

Urinary antiseptic, kidney stones, gout, rheumatism, relief of flatulence and colic, diuretic for edema

- An infusion of the leaves is effective in the treatment of digestive disorders as it soothes the digestive tract and relieves gas. A wonderful cleansing herb, it can relieve chronic kidney problems, stones, and bladder infections. Diuretic, useful for edema and in weight loss to eliminate water.
- The seeds are known to stimulate the pituitary gland, which in turn stimulates the sex hormones to bring on menstruation. It has been used to prevent conception, although when use is stopped, it may increase chances of conceiving as it tones the uterus. Reduces heavy flow and helps with endometriosis.
- The root is slightly bitter but edible, and is rich in Vitamin A. It can be used in a poultice to ease the pain of skin ulcers, or in infusions as a mild laxative, or to expel kidney stones.
- It has been used widely by Indigenous Peoples for pimples, paleness, lack of appetite, to expel intestinal worms, and as a poultice to reduce swelling and soothe sores. An infusion of the blossoms is used to treat diabetes.
- Recent studies using primarily the root show promise in treating several types of cancer, Alzheimer's, cardiovascular disease, and hair loss.

OTHER USES:
- Seeds contain an essential oil used in anti-wrinkle cream.
- A decoction of the seeds and root make a good insecticide.
- Seeds and root can also be used as flavouring for soups and stews.

FOLKLORE: The tiny red flower in the centre is apparently how Queen Anne's Lace got its name, since Queen Anne, according to legend, pricked her finger while making lace. The flower was once believed to cure epilepsy.

INFUSION: Pour 1 cup of boiling water onto 1 tsp. of dried leaves or bruised seeds, infuse 10–15 min. Drink 3 times a day.

TINCTURE: Use 20–60 drops twice a day.

CAUTION: Should not be used by pregnant women as it may stimulate contractions.

RED ALDER

Alnus rubra

Family: Betulaceae

Other names: Oregon Alder, Western Alder, *Fr.* Aulne rouge

Parts used: Inner bark, catkins, leaves, buds

Characteristics: Bitter, cold, dry, stimulating

Systems affected: Liver, large intestine, lymph

Actions: Alterative, anti-inflammatory, antioxidant, astringent, antimicrobial, cathartic, febrifuge, hemostatic, hepatoprotective, emetic, stomachic, tonic

Range: Native to West Coast of British Columbia

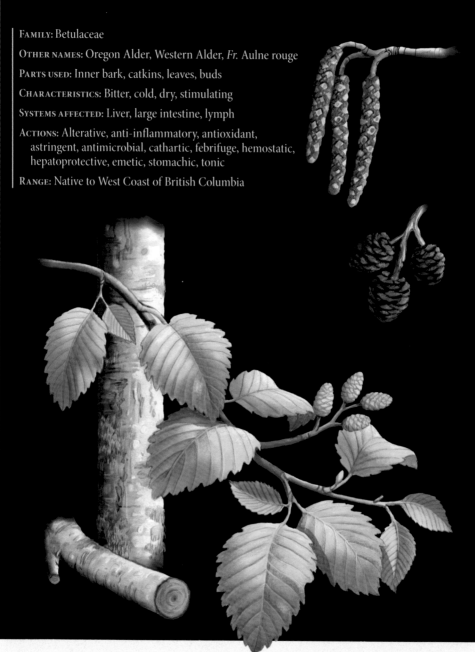

I ndigenous Peoples have used the dried inner bark of this deciduous tree as food and medicine for many years. Native to North America and a member of the birch family, it can grow up to 25 metres tall, and has thin grey or whitish bark often spotted with white patches of lichens or moss. When scraped or cut, the inner bark turns a rusty red colour, giving it its name. The leaves are alternate and toothed, slightly lobed, the edges rolled under. The underside has rusty patches and soft hairs, and the entire leaf turns yellow in the fall. Male flowers or catkins open before the leaves and grow in long, hanging clusters. Female catkins grow on the same branch and are small and cone-like. Near the coast of British Columbia and Alaska it grows mainly on cool and moist slopes; inland, often next to rivers and wetlands. Gather bark in early spring or late autumn, removing no more than a 3–4-inch strip so as not to kill the tree. Dry before using.

MEDICINAL USES:

Pain and headaches, skin problems, digestive sluggishness, hepatitis, diarrhea, lymphatic disorders

- Dried bark used by Indigenous Peoples to treat pain, headaches, rheumatism. Contains salicin, which acts like aspirin, soothing inflammation and relieving pain.
- Alder's bitterness can help support liver function and aid digestion. It stimulates gastric juices, aids bowel function, and increases bile flow. Its tonic action can heal mucous membranes in the digestive tract, decreasing leaky gut, ulcerative colitis, and intestinal bleeding. Inhibits Helicobacter pylori and heals and prevents recurrence of gastric ulcers.
- It can be used both internally and externally for skin problems, such as eczema, boils, pre-menstrual and teen acne, poison oak or ivy, insect bites, scabies, or lice. It helps many chronic or cyclic skin conditions. Inner bark can be ground and used as a poultice or in decoction.
- Decoction useful as a mouthwash for sore throats, gum disease, and thrush.
- Traditionally used for tuberculosis, scrofula, and enlarged lymph nodes. Increases flow of lymph, relieving congestion.
- Used in sitz bath for hemorrhoids and anal fissures.
- Relieves colds and congestion.

OTHER USES:
- Ground inner bark added to soups and bread, catkins high in protein but bitter; used only as survival food.
- Reddish-brown dye made from bark.
- Wood used for furniture.
- Fast-growing and wind-resistant, it helps control erosion and replaces nitrogen in nutrient-poor soil.

DECOCTION: Simmer 1 tsp. dried bark in 1¼ cups water for 10–15 minutes. Let steep for 1 hour, take up to ⅓ cup 4 times a day.

COMBINATIONS:

SKIN: with Sarsaparilla if red and inflamed; with Yellow Dock if oily; with Burdock if dry and flaky; with Elderflower for herpes, eczema, impetigo;

ULCERS: with Licorice, Goldenseal, Yarrow, or Plantain;

LEAKY GUT: with Turmeric, Licorice, or Yarrow.

CAUTION: Avoid use internally if sensitive to aspirin. Use only dried inner bark; fresh bark is emetic.

RED CEDAR

Thuja plicata

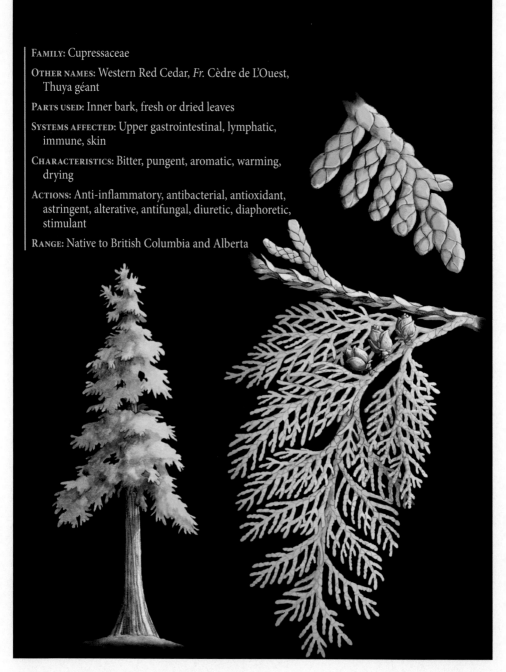

FAMILY: Cupressaceae

OTHER NAMES: Western Red Cedar, *Fr.* Cèdre de L'Ouest, Thuya géant

PARTS USED: Inner bark, fresh or dried leaves

SYSTEMS AFFECTED: Upper gastrointestinal, lymphatic, immune, skin

CHARACTERISTICS: Bitter, pungent, aromatic, warming, drying

ACTIONS: Anti-inflammatory, antibacterial, antioxidant, astringent, alterative, antifungal, diuretic, diaphoretic, stimulant

RANGE: Native to British Columbia and Alberta

The Western Red Cedar has long been considered an important plant to many Indigenous Peoples, holding a sacred place as a symbol of cleansing, protection, and healing. It seems to have an uncanny ability to counteract negative energy. Older trees have been known to reach over 1,000 years of age and can often reach a height of 60 metres and a diameter of 3–5.7 metres; however, overharvesting of trees has left old-growth cedar forests endangered and rare. Its thin, reddish-brown bark is easily peeled off in strips, and the straight trunks flare at the base. The fragrant, fan-shaped groupings of leaves are evergreen, and its name plicata, meaning "plait" or "braid," describes the placement of the leaves on its branches. The inconspicuous pollen cones are located at the tips of the twigs. The seed cones grow to 1–2 cm. with thin, leathery scales, each one bearing one or two winged seeds. Only harvest from freshly fallen branches, as this species is endangered. Hang branches to dry, then chop finely before using.

MEDICINAL USES:

Respiratory tract infections, fevers, colds, kidney problems, rheumatism, skin problems, delayed menstruation, diarrhea, warts

- Hot infusion, steam or tincture of inner bark and/or leaves helps relieve upper respiratory conditions, fevers, coughs, bronchitis; add honey if desired. Good where there is excessive mucous. Stimulates the immune system to fight infection.
- Cold infusion or tincture targets infections in the kidneys and urinary tract.
- Dries oozing skin conditions such as poison oak, eczema, or fungal infections.
- Stimulant properties help relieve sluggishness in digestive, respiratory, urinary, and reproductive systems. A decoction of the bark will induce menstruation.
- Soft pounded bark used to bind open wounds, heal sores, and reduce swelling.
- Decoction from boughs used to help dandruff. Green buds may be chewed to relieve toothache.
- Poultice from crushed bough tips mixed with oil may be applied to the back for coughs, back pain, or rheumatism.

OTHER USES:
- Dried ground inner bark added to flour for making breads.
- Bark used by Indigenous Peoples to make baskets, shredded to make rope and clothing.
- Wood resists decay, often up to a hundred years. Used for building and making canoes, totem poles.
- Offered to sacred fire during sweat lodge ceremonies, burned in smudges, branches boiled to purify the air or to help relieve lung conditions.
- Repels insects, mold, bacteria, and fungi.

INFUSION: 4–6 tbsp. of cold infusion up to 3 times a day

TINCTURE: Fresh leaves 1:2, in 50% alcohol, preferably for topical use only. Should be diluted in water.

COMBINATIONS:

Often used with Witch Hazel to treat eczema. Add Burdock Root or Oregon Grape Root to cool hot skin conditions.

CAUTION: Avoid if pregnant as it can induce menstruation, although steam from simmering Red Cedar may be inhaled to stimulate labour if it is delayed. Contains thujone, a neurotoxin, so prolonged use is not recommended, although short-term use is considered safe. Avoid use of essential oils with infants.

RED CLOVER

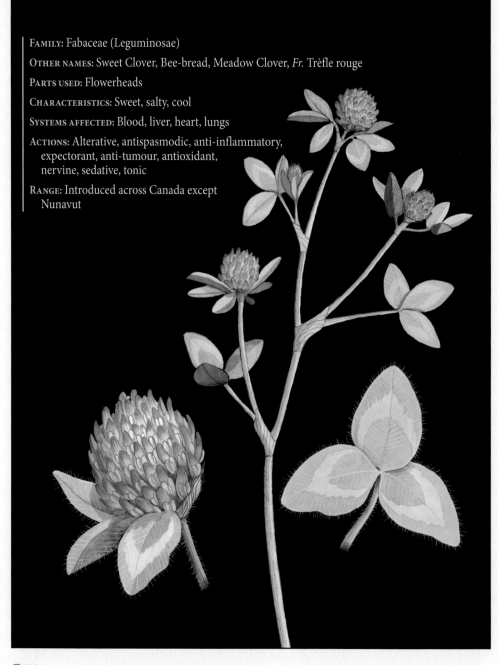

Trifolium pratense

FAMILY: Fabaceae (Leguminosae)

OTHER NAMES: Sweet Clover, Bee-bread, Meadow Clover, *Fr.* Trèfle rouge

PARTS USED: Flowerheads

CHARACTERISTICS: Sweet, salty, cool

SYSTEMS AFFECTED: Blood, liver, heart, lungs

ACTIONS: Alterative, antispasmodic, anti-inflammatory, expectorant, anti-tumour, antioxidant, nervine, sedative, tonic

RANGE: Introduced across Canada except Nunavut

Fields of red clover may be seen across Canada throughout the summer, its sweet scent permeating the air. Originating from Europe, it is often planted by farmers as a cover crop to improve the nitrogen levels in the soil, protect from erosion, and provide feed for animals, but it also grows wild almost everywhere. It is a short-lived perennial, with several stems 30–60 cm. high, arising from the one root and three oval leaflets with a V marked in a lighter green. The flowers are pink or red in a round dense terminal and bloom from June to September. It has been used as a medicinal remedy for centuries, and the young flowerheads, leaves, and sprouts can be eaten. Pick the flowerheads in early summer and dry for later use.

MEDICINAL USES:

Blood thinner, skin diseases, coughs, congestion, fevers, menopause

- Blood purifier and blood thinner, beneficial for thrombosis or thick blood where clots may form.
- Increases elasticity of arteries, and may lower levels of LDL cholesterol, reducing the risk of cardiovascular disease, especially after menopause.
- A rich source of isoflavones, it can mimic estrogen, relieving hot flashes and other discomforts of menopause as well as PMS. Helps prevent bone loss and may improve healing of broken bones.
- Used in salves and liniments for skin complaints, especially in children. For eruptions, psoriasis, eczema, bee stings, etc. Should not be used on open wounds.
- Nlaka'pamux have used an infusion of the blossoms for stomach cancer.
- Effective for coughs, colds, mucous congestion, asthma, bronchitis, whooping cough; the flowers were once dried and smoked to relieve asthma.
- Regulates digestion, improves appetite, increases detoxification ability of the liver.
- Contains several compounds that have anti-cancer properties, and although little clinical research has been done to prove its effectiveness, it appears to limit the growth of cancer by preventing the growth of new blood vessels that feed the tumour.

INFUSION: Pour 1 cup of boiling water onto 1 to 3 tsp. dried flowers. Infuse 10–15 minutes. Take 3 times a day.

COMBINATIONS:

As an alternative, may be combined with Burdock root, Mullein, and Yellow Dock.

CAUTION: Women with hormone-related conditions such as endometriosis, uterine fibroids, breast, ovarian, or uterine cancers, or those using hormonal treatments such as birth control pills or hormone replacement therapy should consult with a professional before taking Red Clover due to the presence of phytoestrogens. Avoid if using blood thinners.

RED ROOT

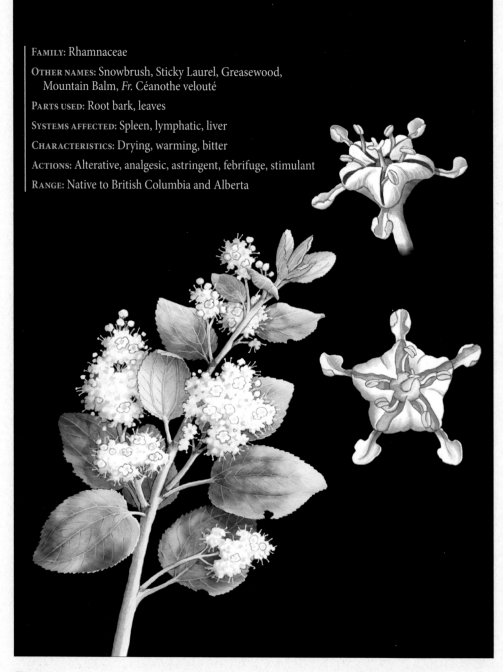

Ceanothus velutinus

FAMILY: Rhamnaceae

OTHER NAMES: Snowbrush, Sticky Laurel, Greasewood, Mountain Balm, *Fr.* Céanothe velouté

PARTS USED: Root bark, leaves

SYSTEMS AFFECTED: Spleen, lymphatic, liver

CHARACTERISTICS: Drying, warming, bitter

ACTIONS: Alterative, analgesic, astringent, febrifuge, stimulant

RANGE: Native to British Columbia and Alberta

Many species of Ceanothus, some of which have similar medicinal uses, grow throughout North America. Here, I will focus on *C. velutinus*, as it is well-known as a medicinal herb and is native to Western Canada, thriving in dry, sunny mid-elevations of the Rockies. An evergreen shrub that grows up to 3 metres, it is often found on land cleared by forest fires, its seeds and roots surviving the devastation. The shiny leaves are identified by 3 prominent veins running from the base to the leaf margins, and are sticky with resin and highly aromatic with a sweet, spicy odour. The small white flowers bloom from June to July and grow in dense clusters which can be smelled metres away. Its central root and thick branches are massive, the inner bark pink to dark red, and rootlets have nodules which fix nitrogen in the soil. The roots may be harvested in mid-summer to early fall by carefully digging up one side and sawing off a branch close to the crown. Fill the hole back in so as not to kill the plant. Peel bark and chop well while still fresh, as it becomes rock-hard and difficult to cut or grind when dried.

MEDICINAL USES:

Congested and swollen lymph glands, indigestion, headaches, fevers, coughs, eczema

- Noted for its action on the lymph nodes, it can loosen stuck fluids, reducing swelling and inflammation. Good for warm swollen glands, tonsillitis, mumps, mononucleosis, pharyngitis, and any catarrhal conditions with a lot of mucous in the lungs or digestive tract. It slowly increases movement and blood flow.
- In Traditional Chinese Medicine, it relieves chronic indigestion due to a congested liver and removes "damp stagnation" from the spleen, characterized by a swollen tongue with a whitish coat, melancholy, sluggishness, poor digestion, constipation, and headache after eating. It opens and restores flow, while the tannins in the root bark tighten and tone tissues and improve assimilation.
- By stimulating blood flow to the brain, it removes brain fog and that "stuck" feeling, when creativity seems blocked.
- Leaves are also used in infusion for fevers and coughs, or as a wash for sores, rashes, or eczema.

OTHER USES:
- Contain saponins, which will produce a lather when mixed with water.
- Flowers and leaves make a nice shampoo.
- Ground leaves can be used as baby powder.

TINCTURE: Dried root bark 1:5, fresh 1:2, in 50% alcohol. Take 30–60 drops up to 5 times a day.

COLD DECOCTION: Take 4–8 tbsp. up to 4 times a day.

COMBINATIONS:

Used mostly with Echinacea for lymph congestion; promotes drainage and fights infection. For liver stagnation with constipation and distention, add Mahonia and Dandelion Root. Other supporting herbs are Calendula, Lobelia, Yarrow, and Mullein.

CAUTION: Avoid use if spleen is inflamed. Do not use while taking blood thinners.

SAGEBRUSH

Artemisia tridentata

FAMILY: Asteraceae

OTHER NAMES: Big Sage, Big Sagebrush, *Fr.* Armoise tridentée

PARTS USED: Leaves, flowers

CHARACTERISTICS: Bitter

ACTIONS: Antirheumatic, antifungal, antiseptic, diaphoretic, digestive, emetic, febrifuge, sedative

RANGE: Native to southern British Columbia and Alberta

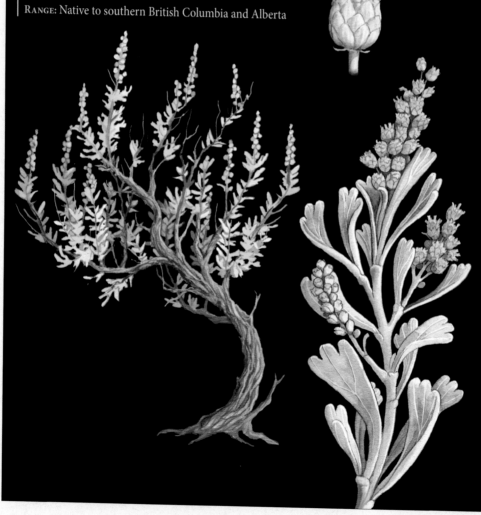

This woody, aromatic evergreen shrub is one of around 150 species of Artemisia in North America, many of which are widely used by Indigenous populations for medicinal and other purposes. Named after the Greek goddess Artemis, it is unrelated to the garden herb Sage, which belongs to the genus Salvia, though its scent is somewhat similar. Usually growing up to around 2 metres high, Sagebrush is mostly found on dry, sunny ranges, deserts, and hillsides, and doesn't tolerate cold temperatures or wet conditions. Its deep taproot has adapted to reach several metres into the soil in search of water. The silvery-grey, wedge-shaped leaves are covered in fine, soft hairs that help it to conserve moisture, and have three teeth at the tip, hence the name tridentata. At the tips of the branches there are clusters of yellow flowers that appear in late summer or early fall. As the bush ages, the bark starts to peel away in fibrous strips that can be used to make ropes or baskets. Harvesting is best done while the plant is in flower. Strip away small stems and leaves from mature plants, wash to remove dust and hang upside down to dry. They will keep for about 2 years.

MEDICINAL USES:

Fungal infections, arthritis, parasites, colds, coughs, congestion, fevers, digestive problems, diarrhea

- Contains thujone, making it antimicrobial and antiparasitic; however, it needs to be used with caution as it can be toxic if taken internally in large doses. Used to treat worms and food- and water-borne illnesses such as salmonella and amoebic infections (traveller's diarrhea).
- Applied topically for wounds and ulcers as well as fungal infections such as ringworm or athlete's foot. Relieves pain from sprains or chronic diseases like arthritis. May be used in compresses or by applying wet leaves as a poultice.
- A tea or decoction is bitter-tasting but can be sipped slowly to help digestive upsets, clear mucous in coughs, bronchitis, and colds, and promote sweating to relieve fever. When mixed with salt and used as a gargle it can help sore throats.
- Steam from boiling the herb can relieve headaches and clear sinus congestion. Infused oil is used for chest congestion and sprains.
- Brings on menstruation.

OTHER USES:
- Leaves and buds produce a yellow dye.
- Bark fibre used to make mats, baskets, rope, and to stuff pillows.
- Leaves and branches used as a ceremonial smudge for purification.
- Seeds can be eaten raw or dried or ground into meal.

COLD INFUSION: 2–4 tbsp. up to 3 times a day.

CAUTION: Do not use if pregnant or nursing. Discontinue use if dizziness, nausea, or headache occur. Toxic if taken in large doses or over a long period of time. Do not use for more than 1 week consecutively.

SEA BUCKTHORN

Hippophae rhamnoides

FAMILY: Elaeagnaceae

OTHER NAMES: Siberian Pineapple, Sandthorn, Seaberry, Sallowthorn, *Fr.* Argousier

PARTS USED: Whole plant, mainly berries, leaves, seeds

SYSTEMS AFFECTED: Cardiovascular, digestive, skin

CHARACTERISTICS: Acidic, astringent

ACTIONS: Anti-inflammatory, antimicrobial, antiviral, antihypertensive, hepatoprotective, neuroprotective, tonic

RANGE: Introduced in the Yukon, Alberta, Saskatchewan, Ontario, Quebec

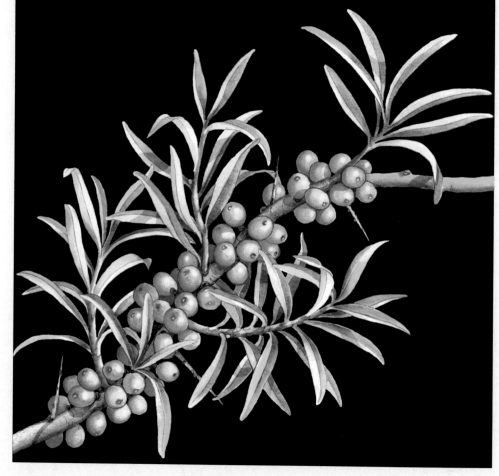

Originating in China, Tibet, and the Himalayas, this attractive deciduous shrub was introduced into Europe and North America for its abundant nutritive and medicinal properties. Usually found growing in coastal areas, it is often used to help erosion, and it improves soil quality by fixing nitrogen through its root nodules. It prefers moist but not boggy conditions and can tolerate salt spray, but it's a hardy plant that will grow in poor soil as long as there is full sun. Its bright orange berries are used around the world for their oil, mostly in skin products, but recent studies have shown that it may have potential for its ability to help with other conditions, from ulcers to heart disease and even cancer, although more research is needed. Growing to around 8 metres high or even larger in some countries, it has silvery-green, lance-shaped leaves and thorny branches. Male and female plants are separate, and both are needed to produce berries, which grow in dense clumps along the branches. Each berry produces one shiny brown seed, usually in September or October. Fruit is usually harvested before the first frost, but must be done with care due to the thorns and the fact that they don't let go easily. Use a pair of pruning shears to remove one by one or simply snip off a branch and freeze, as the berries come away easier when frozen. Be careful not to overharvest, as you can kill the plant, and only prune every second year to give it time to recover.

MEDICINAL USES:

Ulcers, digestive problems, liver injury, high cholesterol, skin diseases, cancer, obesity, joint inflammation

- Very nutrient-rich, the berries contain vitamins A, B12, C, E, riboflavin, niacin, phosphorus, potassium, calcium, magnesium, iron, amino acids, lutein, and omega fatty acids. Used in the food industry to boost nutrients in food or juices.
- Balances oil levels on the skin and scalp, reducing acne and inflammation. Improves elasticity, repairs free-radical injury from sunburn, helps eczema, psoriasis, dermatitis, dryness in the vagina. May be taken orally and/or topically.
- Lubricates and repairs the mucous membrane of the intestinal tract, improves slow digestion, gastric ulcers.
- Protects cardiovascular system, lowers cholesterol, thins the blood.
- Shows promise in treatment of some cancers, particularly colon and stomach cancer and in prevention of prostate cancer, but more research is needed.
- May have an effect on obesity by reducing the appetite and improving the gut microbiome.
- Helps repair liver injuries and inflammation.
- Its neuroprotective properties may prove promising in treatment of Alzheimer's disease.
- Taking an oil supplement may reduce symptoms of dry eyes and reddening.
- Branches and leaves also produce an oil used for burn ointments.

CAUTION: No known toxicity, may slightly lower blood pressure. Thins the blood; avoid using within 2 weeks of surgery or if taking blood-thinning medication. Avoid during pregnancy. May cause yellowing of the skin if used over a long period of time.

SENECA SNAKEROOT

Polygala senega

FAMILY: Polygalaceae

OTHER NAMES: Milkwort, Mountain Flax, Rattlesnake Root, Senega Root, *Fr.* Polygale sénéca, Polygale de Virginie

PARTS USED: Root, aerial

CHARACTERISTICS: Bitter, acidic

SYSTEMS AFFECTED: Upper and lower gastrointestinal, respiratory, parasympathetic

ACTIONS: Anti-inflammatory, cathartic, diuretic, diaphoretic, emetic, emmenagogue, expectorant, stimulant

RANGE: Native to southern British Columbia, Alberta, Saskatchewan, Manitoba, Ontario, Quebec, New Brunswick

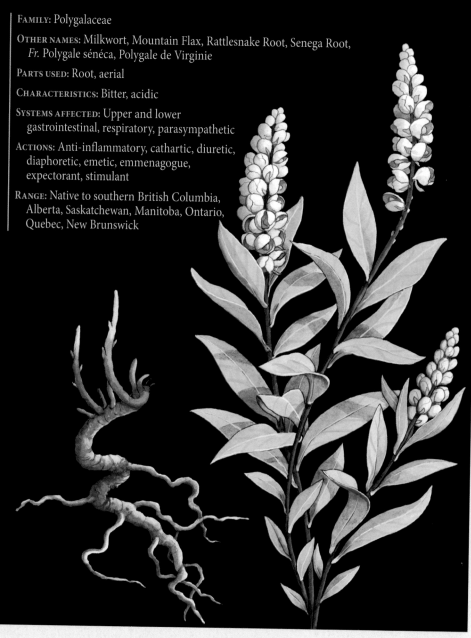

As its name suggests, this plant was originally used as a remedy for snakebites by Indigenous Peoples, specifically the Seneca Nation living just south of Lake Ontario. Up until the 1950s, Indigenous Peoples in Manitoba grew and harvested three quarters of the world's supply, exporting to Europe, Japan, and the US as an effective cough remedy. Since the discovery of synthetic replacements, the market has somewhat decreased, although it is still popular with herbalists. This small perennial from the Milkwort family grows from 15–40 cm. tall, thriving on rocky soils, woodlands, prairies, and abandoned fields across Canada, although mostly absent from NS, PEI, and NL. Leaves are lance-shaped and alternate along the vertical stems sprouting from the rootstock, becoming small and scale-like towards the bottom of the stem. The white, pinkish, or greenish flowers bloom in late June or July, looking very much like the rattle of a rattlesnake atop the unbranched stem, each flower having a bud-like appearance, even in full bloom. The root is twisted and snake-like, taking at least four years to grow large enough to use as medicine. There is a distinctive ridge on one side, and the odour and taste are pretty disagreeable, although that diminishes as it dries. The best time to harvest is in the fall, although it's best to mark the plants while still in bloom so they can be identified later.

MEDICINAL USES:

Snakebites, respiratory problems, earaches, rheumatism, amenorrhea

- Contains triterpenoid saponins which produce a soap-like foam when mixed with water. This irritates the gastric mucosa and causes secretion of mucous in the bronchioles, breaking up phlegm and reducing its viscosity. Used for deep, rattling coughs with excessive excretions such as chronic bronchitis, bronchopneumonia, bronchial asthma, laryngitis, whooping cough and pleurisy.
- Traditionally used by Indigenous Peoples for snakebite by chewing the root and placing the pulp over the wound. Root used by the Cree as a toothache remedy, and the juice swallowed for colds and sore throats.
- Brings on menstruation; uterine stimulant.
- Emetic and cathartic (laxative) when taken in large doses.
- Some research has shown it to be effective in reducing cancer cell growth, specifically in lung cancer.

TINCTURE: Fresh 1:2, dry 1:5, 65% alcohol. Take 10–45 drops up to 4 times a day, depending on how much is tolerated. Small, frequent doses work best to avoid nausea.

DECOCTION: Boil 2 tbsp. dried root in 3 cups water, reduce to 2 cups. Take 1 tbsp. at a time at 1-hour intervals.

CAUTION: Do not exceed recommended dose; may cause violent vomiting and diarrhea. Do not use if pregnant or lactating or if you have peptic ulcers or inflammatory bowel disease.

SHEPHERD'S PURSE

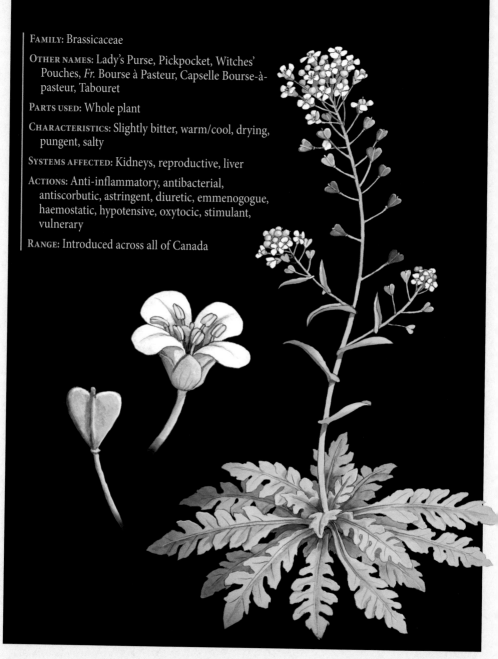

Capsella bursa-pastoris

FAMILY: Brassicaceae

OTHER NAMES: Lady's Purse, Pickpocket, Witches' Pouches, *Fr.* Bourse à Pasteur, Capselle Bourse-à-pasteur, Tabouret

PARTS USED: Whole plant

CHARACTERISTICS: Slightly bitter, warm/cool, drying, pungent, salty

SYSTEMS AFFECTED: Kidneys, reproductive, liver

ACTIONS: Anti-inflammatory, antibacterial, antiscorbutic, astringent, diuretic, emmenogogue, haemostatic, hypotensive, oxytocic, stimulant, vulnerary

RANGE: Introduced across all of Canada

This common annual or biennial weed originated in Europe but is now found in most corners of the world. It usually grows to a height of 30–60 cm., preferring cultivated soil, gardens, and waste places that get sun most of the day. A member of the cabbage, mustard, and broccoli family, it is distinguished by its flat, green, heart-shaped fruits growing along the flower stalk which emerges from a rosette of lobed basal leaves about 23 cm. across and resembles that of a dandelion without the milky sap. The tiny white 4-petalled flowers grow in terminal clusters on the erect stem and are replaced by the heart-shaped seedpods. Below the flowers and seedpods are small arrow-shaped leaves clasping the stem. Harvest the plants in the summer and use fresh, or dry for later use. Should be used within 1 year as it quickly loses its potency.

MEDICINAL USES:

Bleeding, childbirth, cancer, urinary calculus, menorrhagia, cystitis, hemorrhoids

- Infusion or tincture used for all kinds of internal bleeding or hemorrhage in the stomach, lungs, uterus, or kidneys. Leaves can be mashed, mixed with hot water, and applied as a poultice to bruises. Leaves can be bruised and applied directly to wounds to staunch bleeding. For nosebleeds, soak a cotton ball in infusion and insert into the nostril.
- Has proven uterine-contracting properties. Used during childbirth to aid labour, tone the uterus after childbirth, and reduce bleeding. Not for use during pregnancy as it may provoke miscarriage. Helps prevent prolapse of the uterus. Constricts smooth muscles surrounding the blood vessels, especially in the uterus; improves clotting.
- Helps PMS, and stops heavy menstrual bleeding due to fibroids, endometriosis, IUDs, and chronic menorrhagia.
- Has long been a folk remedy for cancer, and has been proven effective at reducing growth of Ehrlich tumours in mice.
- Helps remove urinary stones, abscesses, and ulcers in the bladder, and can be used for cystitis and blood in the urine.
- Remedy for diarrhea, dysentery, and bleeding hemorrhoids. Tones the tissues, prevents atrophy of the muscles in the digestive tract, uterus, and bladder, tones and strengthens.
- Contains vitamins A, C, K, iron, calcium and omega-3 fatty acids. Best if picked before flowering. Leaves eaten raw in salads or cooked if older, as they become more peppery with age.

OTHER USES:
- Seeds placed in water attract mosquitoes and stick to their mouths.
- Toxic to mosquito larvae.
- Often planted on marshy land to absorb the salt and improve soil quality for gardening.

TINCTURE: Fresh 1:2, recently dried 1:5, in 50% alcohol. (Note: tincture may take on a funky smell; this is normal). Take 20–60 drops at intervals throughout the day. Stop taking when it starts working.

INFUSION: 1–2 tsp. dried herb in 1 cup hot water. Steep 15 min., strain and cool. Take 2–3 times per day.

COMBINATIONS:

May be used with Lady's Mantle, and Raspberry leaf for heavy periods. With Licorice root, it has a strong antibacterial effect against oral infections.

CAUTION: Causes uterine contractions; do not take during pregnancy. Use with caution if there is a pre-existing heart condition. Do not use for at least 2 weeks prior to surgery as it may interact with anesthesia.

SKULLCAP

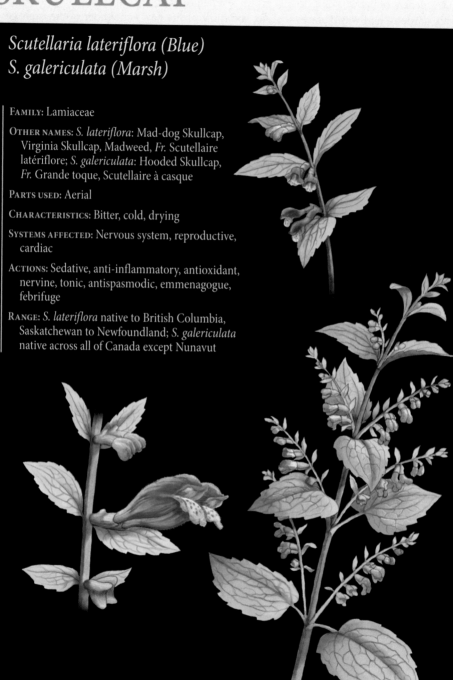

Scutellaria lateriflora (Blue)
S. galericulata (Marsh)

FAMILY: Lamiaceae

OTHER NAMES: *S. lateriflora*: Mad-dog Skullcap, Virginia Skullcap, Madweed, *Fr.* Scutellaire latériflore; *S. galericulata*: Hooded Skullcap, *Fr.* Grande toque, Scutellaire à casque

PARTS USED: Aerial

CHARACTERISTICS: Bitter, cold, drying

SYSTEMS AFFECTED: Nervous system, reproductive, cardiac

ACTIONS: Sedative, anti-inflammatory, antioxidant, nervine, tonic, antispasmodic, emmenagogue, febrifuge

RANGE: *S. lateriflora* native to British Columbia, Saskatchewan to Newfoundland; *S. galericulata* native across all of Canada except Nunavut

A perennial plant native to North America, Skullcap has been used for centuries by Indigenous Peoples due to its effectiveness in treating nervous disorders and menstrual problems. It prefers partially shaded wetland areas and its erect square stem grows to a height of 45–60 cm. with occasional branches. It has broad, lance-shaped, toothed leaves in opposite pairs, and from July to September bears blue-lavender, two-lipped, tube-shaped flowers, the upper lip forming a hood, the lower having two lobes, somewhat resembling a helmet or cap. *S. lateriflora* is easily identified by a protuberance on the upper calyx. It should not be confused with the Chinese variety (*Scutellaria baicalensis* or Huang qin), which has different medicinal properties. Skullcap should be harvested while the flowers are in full bloom and dried for future use, although better used fresh in making tinctures if possible.

MEDICINAL USES:

Nervous disorders, insomnia, epilepsy, suppressed menstruation

- Tonic and restorative properties help nourish the nervous system. It relaxes nervous tension during prolonged periods of stress, calms, promotes sleep, and eases anxiety, busy mind, and panic attacks. Effects are accumulative and it may be used over long periods of time. Not a strong sedative but may be combined with other herbs like Valerian for sleep.
- Eases PMS symptoms, promotes menstruation.
- Indigenous Peoples traditionally use it as a tea for heart problems, ulcers and fevers.
- Contains scutellarin, a flavonoid with antispasmodic properties, used for epilepsy, convulsions, and spasms.
- Helps with alcohol and drug withdrawal, lessens the severity of symptoms and detoxifies.
- Eases the symptoms of neuralgia and fibromyalgia.
- Relieves incessant coughing and pneumonia.
- Reduces fever, increases blood flow, lessens inflammation.
- Best when used on "hot" or "type A" personalities; that is, easily overheated and excited, with a red tongue and fast pulse.

FOLKLORE: In the eighteenth century it was claimed to be a cure for rabies, hence the names Mad Dog and Madweed, but this was soon discredited, although it does relieve some of the symptoms.

INFUSION: 1 cup hot water to 1 tsp. dried herb or 2 tsp. fresh, infuse 15 minutes. Drink 3 times a day. Should not be boiled.

TINCTURE: Take 1–2 ml. 3 times a day.

COMBINATIONS:

For insomnia, may be combined with Valerian root, Lemon Balm, Chamomile or Passionflower.

CAUTION: Do not take during pregnancy as it may cause miscarriage. Do not exceed recommended doses as it may cause confusion, stupor, irregular heartbeat, and twitching, and in rare cases liver toxicity.

SORREL

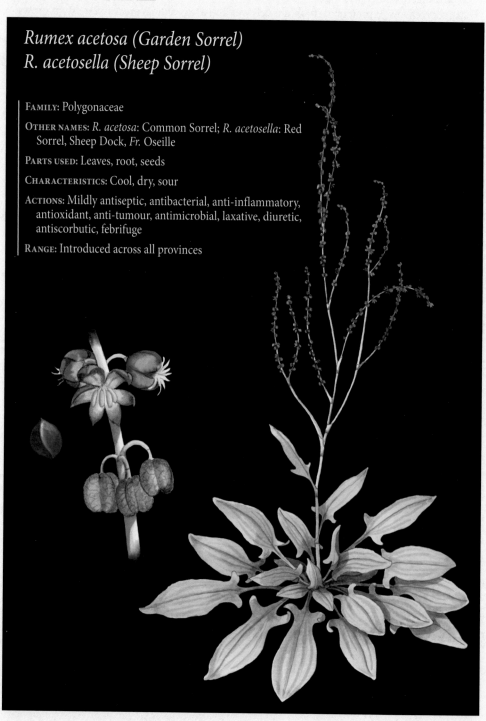

Rumex acetosa (Garden Sorrel)
R. acetosella (Sheep Sorrel)

FAMILY: Polygonaceae

OTHER NAMES: *R. acetosa*: Common Sorrel; *R. acetosella*: Red Sorrel, Sheep Dock, *Fr.* Oseille

PARTS USED: Leaves, root, seeds

CHARACTERISTICS: Cool, dry, sour

ACTIONS: Mildly antiseptic, antibacterial, anti-inflammatory, antioxidant, anti-tumour, antimicrobial, laxative, diuretic, antiscorbutic, febrifuge

RANGE: Introduced across all provinces

This common perennial originating from Europe grows abundantly in meadows, pastures, and backyards throughout Canada and has been used around the world for centuries in salads, as a vegetable and as a potherb. It has a sharp, tangy taste due to the presence of oxalic acid, and is loaded with nutrients, including vitamins A and C, iron, magnesium, potassium, and calcium. Garden Sorrel often grows up to 60 cm. high; it branches at the top, its leaves are 10–15 cm. long and shaped like an arrowhead. The dark red or purplish flower spikes stand out in a field of grasses and turn into reddish-brown seedpods in the fall. *R. acetosella* is very similar to *R. acetosa* except it grows to about 40 cm. and the leaves are from 2.5–7.6 cm. long. Leaves are best harvested early in the summer when they are tender.

MEDICINAL USES:

Fevers, inflammation, cancer, sinusitis, type 2 diabetes, hemorrhoids, skin irritations

- Leaves can be eaten raw in mixed salads, cooked in stews, or eaten like spinach. Perfectly safe in moderate quantities, but due to the presence of oxalic acid, should not be consumed in excessive amounts raw; when cooking large amounts, change the water halfway through the process to remove the oxalic acid. Use only a stainless steel or glass pot, as other metals may affect the taste.
- Infusion used as a diuretic, as an appetite stimulant, for treating kidney stones, to reduce fever, and to soothe an upset stomach.
- Root and seed traditionally used as an astringent to stop hemorrhage.
- The juice from the leaves is used as a gargle for mouth ulcers, in a compress to treat cysts, heal wounds and itching, staunch bleeding, reduce swelling, and inflammation. It makes a cooling drink for fevers.
- Improves digestion and provides nutrients and antioxidants which can prevent cancer, lower blood pressure, and improve the condition of diabetics. Sheep Sorrel is a key ingredient in the formula for Essiac Tea, a herbal formula which may have some potent antioxidant and DNA-protective activity in the treatment of some cancers.

OTHER USES:
- Roots and stems are used to obtain dyes.
- The juice is sometimes used to remove stains from linen.

INFUSION: Standard. Drink 20–30 ml. up to twice a day.

CAUTION: Since the presence of oxalic acid is quite high, it is inadvisable to consume in large quantities, particularly if you have a history of kidney stones.

SPRUCE

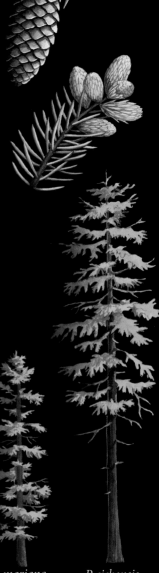

Picea engelmannii (Mountain Spruce)
P. sitchensis (Sitka Spruce)
P. glauca (White Spruce)
P. mariana (Black Spruce)

FAMILY: Pinaceae

OTHER NAMES: *P. engelmannii*: Silver Spruce, Engelmann Spruce, *Fr.* Épinette d'Engelmann; *P. sitchensis*: Coast Spruce, Tideland Spruce, *Fr.* Épinette de Sitka; *P. glauca*: Canadian Spruce, Skunk Spruce, *Fr.* Épinette blanche; *P. mariana*: *Fr.* Épinette noir

PARTS USED: Pitch (resin), young tips, needles, cones

SYSTEMS AFFECTED: Skin, urinary, respiratory

ACTIONS: Antiseptic, analgesic, antifungal, carminative, diaphoretic, diuretic, expectorant, laxative

RANGE: *P. engelmannii* native to British Columbia and Alberta; *P. sitchensis* native to British Columbia coast; *P. glauca* native across all of Canada; *P. mariana* native across all of Canada

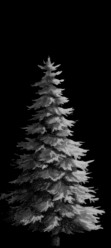

P. glauca

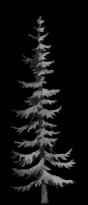

P. engelmannii

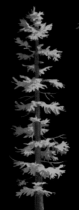

P. mariana

P. sichensis

Spruce trees are one of the most common trees in Canada, found everywhere except for the northernmost regions. They are identified by their 4-sided, short, pointed needles arranged in spirals around the stem. Unlike Pine needles, which grow in clusters, Spruce needles grow singularly on small peg-like projections that remain when the needles fall, usually every four to ten years. The bark is scaly and cones hang downward after pollination. Indigenous Peoples rely heavily on this tree, not only as medicine, but for building materials, food, basket-making, and many other uses. The slow-growing Mountain Spruce is slender and conical, found in the high altitudes of BC and Alberta and averaging about 30 metres in height. The Sitka Spruce, on the other hand, grows more slowly but is the largest Spruce, sometimes reaching heights of up to 90 metres, with few branches lower than 30 metres. White and Black Spruce grow across Canada and are usually under 30 metres tall. The former smells a bit skunky and has shallow roots that make them prone to blowing over in a bad windstorm. Harvest Spruce tips in the spring as soon as the papery sheath falls off. Ideally, cool them within a few hours of harvest as they can get hot and cook themselves if left in a bag for too long.

MEDICINAL USES:

Wounds, coughs, sore throat, colds, rheumatism, muscle pain

- Small bright green tips are rich in Vitamins A and C and potassium, have a pleasant aroma, and make a nice tea for coughs, colds, or flu, or can be made into jellies, glazes for meat, mixed into stuffings, or added as a pot herb. Used as a spring tonic.
- Decoction of needles and cones can be used as a wash for rashes, hives, burns, or as tea for colds, sore throat, or gargled for gum problems and toothache. The Nlaka'pamux use a decoction of needles and resin taken directly from the bark blisters to treat cancer, coughs.
- Resin or pitch is antiseptic and analgesic, can be applied to wounds or warmed and smeared on a piece of cloth, which is then warmed in the oven and applied to chest for coughs or back for backache. Boil resin in water for urinary or digestive problems.
- Ointment or infused oil made from resin can be applied to sore joints and muscles to relieve pain, or to insect bites, chapped hands, eczema, burns, or rashes.

OTHER USES:
- Roots peeled and split for making ropes, baskets, and hats.
- Inner bark used as emergency food, or ground into meal and added to flour.
- Softened pitch used to waterproof boats; wood used for building, making canoes, snowshoes, and utensils, and it has acoustic properties for making pianos and guitars.
- Fresh shoots used to make spruce beer.

DECOCTION: Break several branches into small pieces and add with cones to 17 cups of water. Bring to a boil and simmer 20 minutes. Breathe in vapours for congestion or drink for colds and flu. Sip 2–3 tsp. 3 or 4 times a day.

FERMENTED SYRUP: Macerate the tips in cane sugar for a number of months to develop the flavours. Strain and can or freeze.

CAUTION: Best when used in acute conditions over a short term and in small doses. Avoid during pregnancy.

STINGING NETTLE

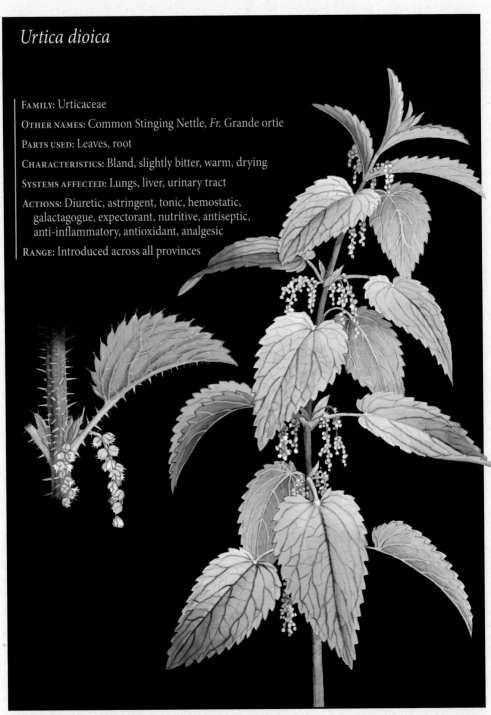

Urtica dioica

FAMILY: Urticaceae

OTHER NAMES: Common Stinging Nettle, *Fr.* Grande ortie

PARTS USED: Leaves, root

CHARACTERISTICS: Bland, slightly bitter, warm, drying

SYSTEMS AFFECTED: Lungs, liver, urinary tract

ACTIONS: Diuretic, astringent, tonic, hemostatic, galactagogue, expectorant, nutritive, antiseptic, anti-inflammatory, antioxidant, analgesic

RANGE: Introduced across all provinces

Although these plants have a bad reputation for their stinging hairs, if properly handled they are one of the best medicinal herbs, with a wide variety of applications. A perennial which grows from 30–90 cm. high, it has oval leaves which are opposite, tapered to a point, and finely toothed. The roots are creeping rhizomes, so it multiplies easily. The flowers are greenish and hang in branched clusters. The stiff hairs covering the entire plant contain a small amount of formic acid, which give its sting, but it can be neutralized by rubbing Dock leaf or Plantain onto affected areas. It loses its sting after it's been dried or cooked or even stored in the refrigerator for a day or so. It is usually found in waste places and ditches where the soil is moist; gather with rubber gloves in the spring or early summer when the leaves are free of dew, and hang to dry in a shaded area for later use.

MEDICINAL USES:

Arthritis, asthma, bronchitis, eczema, cystitis, stagnant mucous, enlarged prostate, stones, diarrhea, hemorrhoids, hay fever

- Makes a wonderful spring tonic, cleansing herb, and blood purifier, high in vitamins C and A, potassium, protein, and iron. The young leaves steamed taste like spinach and when eaten over a long period can benefit those with anemia or depleted energy from loss of fluids. Also, when steamed for 30 minutes, the juice may be squeezed out and 1 tbsp. taken every hour can reduce PMS, heavy menstruation, and stop bleeding.
- After childbirth, nettle tea may be used to promote milk production and build up the blood. Combines well with Raspberry leaf for this purpose.
- Contains a high amount of sterols, especially in the root, and may be effective in treating enlarged prostate or Benign Prostatic Hypertrophy and stimulating the white blood cells to counteract inflammation.
- Removes stagnant mucous in the lungs and sinuses; useful for asthma, pneumonia, pleurisy, bronchitis, and allergies. Traditionally it was burned and the smoke inhaled for lung infections.
- Useful for lowering uric acid levels, it can prevent or treat gout and kidney or bladder stones. Good for urinary tract infections.
- Relieves diarrhea, dysentery, hemorrhoids, mucous in the stool, or any cold, damp conditions.
- Compresses reduce pain of arthritis, rheumatism. Purposefully stinging oneself causes increased blood flow to the skin, relieving inflammation of the joints.

OTHER USES: Fibres used to make fabrics and clothing, rope, netting.

INFUSION: Mix 1–3 tsp. dried herb in 1 cup boiling water; infuse 10–15 min. Drink as needed.

TINCTURE: Standard, 1–4 ml. 3 times a day.

CAUTION: Handle with gloves. Not recommended for pregnant women. Could interfere with blood-thinning drugs or diuretic drugs. May lower blood pressure. Do not apply to open wounds.

ST. JOHN'S WORT

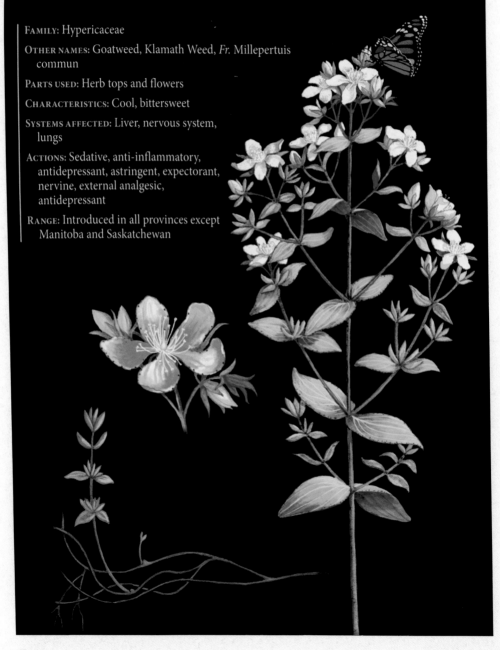

Hypericum perforatum

Family: Hypericaceae

Other names: Goatweed, Klamath Weed, *Fr.* Millepertuis commun

Parts used: Herb tops and flowers

Characteristics: Cool, bittersweet

Systems affected: Liver, nervous system, lungs

Actions: Sedative, anti-inflammatory, antidepressant, astringent, expectorant, nervine, external analgesic, antidepressant

Range: Introduced in all provinces except Manitoba and Saskatchewan

Waterpepper or Smartweed is just one of a large family of similar weeds growing throughout North America. It is an annual native to Europe that grows in damp muddy areas, ditches, and along riverbanks, and has a bitter peppery taste. It can reach 30–50 cm. in height with branched stems and dark green, lance-shaped leaves with undulate edges and glands on the underside. The tiny pink or greenish flowers are arranged on terminal spikes, and the fruit is triangular, flat, and dark brown. It is harvested in summer during flowering and dried in the shade, but is more potent if used fresh.

MEDICINAL USES:

Nervous system disorders, depression, anxiety, viral infections, arthritic pain

- Primarily used today to relieve symptoms of anxiety and mild to moderate depression, it also helps with SAD, PMS, menopause, and insomnia due to the presence of hyperforin, which calms the nervous system. It could take 1–3 months before you see results.
- May be effective in easing nerve pain, lower back pain, rheumatism, arthritis, and chronic inflammation.
- An oil or ointment made from the flowers has been used since the Middle Ages as an astringent to heal wounds, sores, bruises, burns, insect bites, and hemorrhoids and to help prevent inflammation.
- Used traditionally by Indigenous Peoples as a tea to protect against tuberculosis and other respiratory ailments, as well as for fever, diarrhea, snakebite, and skin problems.
- Contains hypericin, which has been proven an effective antiviral in the treatment of HIV/AIDS, herpes, hepatitis, and several types of cancer.
- A cup of infusion before bed can help children with bedwetting.

FOLKLORE: Named after St. John the Baptist, as it usually flowers around June 24, St. John's Day. In Ancient Greece its fragrance was believed to chase away evil spirits, and was used for centuries as a charm against witchcraft and in exorcisms. In medieval times, women would pick the herb on St. John's Eve with the dew still on the leaves; it was believed this would help them find a husband.

INFUSION: Add 1–2 tsp. herb to 1 cup boiling water, steep 10–15 minutes, drink up to 3 times a day.

TINCTURE: Take 1–4 ml of tincture 3 times a day.

OIL: Place flowers in a glass jar and add enough olive oil just to cover. Place jar in a sunny window for 2–3 weeks, shaking daily. Filter and place in dark glass container.

CAUTION: Excessive use may cause photosensitivity or allergies in some people. Do not take in combination with other drugs, narcotics, alcohol, cold or hay fever medications, birth control pills, tryptophan, or tyrosine. Do not use during pregnancy.

SUBALPINE FIR

Abies lasiocarpa
A. balsamea (Balsam Fir)

FAMILY: Pinaceae

OTHER NAMES: *A. lasiocarpa*: Mountain Balsam Fir, Alpine Fir, White Fir, Rocky Mountain Fir, *Fr.* Sapin de montagne, Sapin concolore; *A. balsamea*: *Fr.* Sapin Baumier

PARTS USED: Resin, needles, bark

ACTIONS: Antioxidant, antiseptic, antifungal, diuretic, expectorant, diaphoretic, laxative, tonic

RANGE: *A. lasiocarpa* native to British Columbia, Southern Yukon, Alberta; *A. balsamea* native from Alberta to Newfoundland

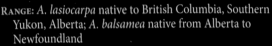

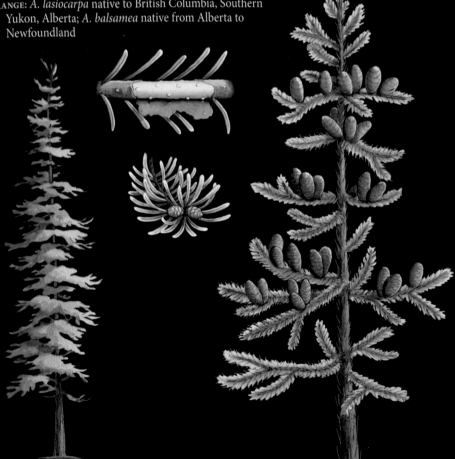

Known as the "Medicine Tree" by some Indigenous Peoples, the Subalpine Fir has been a traditional medicine for lung ailments for centuries. This native evergreen is the smallest of the true firs, growing up to 50 metres in height, but usually smaller, and shrub-like close to the timberline. Mostly found above 600 metres, it prefers the higher elevations but can occasionally be found along the coastline, its short, rigid branches making it look more slender and spire-like than other conifers. The needles are about 2.5 cm. long, soft, flat, and blunt or sometimes notched at the tip, usually curving upwards. The dark purple cones stand upward on the branch and often have globs of pitch stuck to them, which tend to drip when the weather gets warm. The grey, smooth bark on young trees has resin blisters, but as the trees get older the bark becomes cracked and fissured, with reddish scales. Balsam Fir needles tend to lie flatter than the Subalpine Fir, but is otherwise very similar. Bark and needles can be harvested at any time, but the vitamin C content is higher in the winter.

MEDICINAL USES:

Colds and flu, fever, lung ailments, insomnia, wounds, burns

- Antiseptic and analgesic, the resin from blisters on the bark may be applied to wounds, sores, and burns. Speeds healing.
- Decoction of bark and needles is high in vitamin C, works as a tonic for colds and flu, lung ailments, fevers, and trouble sleeping. Poultice of needles can be applied to the chest for coughs and chest colds and to induce sweating.
- Pitch can be chewed to clean the teeth, or made into an infusion for gargling for a sore throat or bad breath. May be emetic if taken internally.

OTHER USES:
- Cones may be ground to a powder, mixed with fat, and eaten as a snack. Aids digestion.
- Inner bark can be dried, ground, and mixed with flour for bread-making.
- An infusion made from the needles can be used as a deodorant.
- Boughs often strewn onto floors of teepees or sweat lodges or burned as incense in ceremonies.
- Powdered needles mixed with bear grease to make a pleasant-smelling hair tonic, and to help dandruff.
- An aromatic massage oil can be made by infusing needles in olive oil for 4–6 weeks and then straining.

DECOCTION: Break up branches and put into a pot, cover with water, and bring to a boil, simmer for 20 minutes until the aroma fills the room. Breathe in steam. Once liquid has cooled slightly, strain into a container. Drink 2–3 cups a day. Add honey if desired.

CAUTION: Pitch can induce vomiting in strong doses. May cause skin reactions in some people. Use in moderation.

THIMBLEBERRY

Rubus parviflorus
R. idaeus (Raspberry)

FAMILY: Rosaceae

OTHER NAMES: Redcap, Western Thimbleberry, White
Flowering Raspberry, *Fr.* Ronce à petites fleurs

PARTS USED: Berries, leaves, bark

SYSTEMS AFFECTED: Spleen, liver, kidneys, reproductive

CHARACTERISTICS: Leaves: Bitter, cool; berries: tart/sweet

ACTIONS: Antiemetic, astringent, blood tonic, hemostatic,
parturient, stomachic

RANGE: *R. parviflorus* native to British Columbia, Alberta,
Southern Ontario; *R. idaeus* native across all of Canada

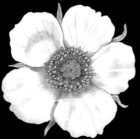

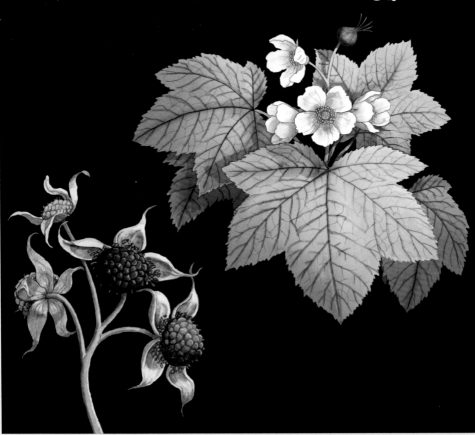

This deciduous shrub closely resembles the common Raspberry; however, there are a few differences. The fruit when picked has a wider cavity, large enough to insert a finger, much like a thimble. Also, there are no prickles on the stems or leaves, only very fine hairs that give the leaves a downy feel, making them useful as a toilet paper substitute in an emergency. The leaves are toothed and shaped like a maple leaf, usually wider than they are long, with 5 lobes and lighter green on the underside. The white flowers appear in June, have a yellow centre, and grow in clusters of 2 to 7. The fruit ripens later in the summer, going from white to pink to red, and tastes a little more tart than a Raspberry. The bark sheds in tiny pieces and canes are biennial, with flowers appearing in the second year. It grows in thickets, is shade tolerant, and can thrive in moist or fairly dry soils. Pick leaves when the plant is in flower and hang to dry in the shade for later use.

MEDICINAL USES:

Wounds, acne, nausea, diarrhea, menorrhagia, childbirth, lack of appetite

- Berries are high in vitamins C and A, used to treat scurvy and build immunity.
- A poultice of dried or fresh leaves treats wounds, burns, and acne, helping to prevent scarring.
- A decoction made from the roots is used as a treatment for nausea, vomiting, diarrhea, and dysentery.
- Infusion of leaves can reduce heavy periods and tone the uterine muscles, reducing inflammation and swelling. Prepares the uterus for childbirth and helps speed recovery afterwards.
- Root tea increases appetite, tones and strengthens the stomach.

OTHER USES: Young shoots can be eaten in salads or steamed as a vegetable.

INFUSION: Standard, 6–8 ounces 3 times a day.

CAUTION: Avoid using wilted leaves, only fresh or dried. Berries can irritate the colon if you have diverticulosis.

VALERIAN

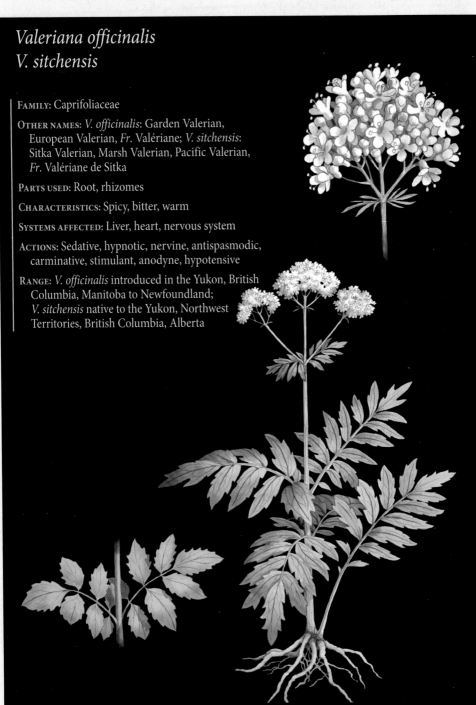

Valeriana officinalis
V. sitchensis

FAMILY: Caprifoliaceae

OTHER NAMES: *V. officinalis*: Garden Valerian, European Valerian, *Fr.* Valériane; *V. sitchensis*: Sitka Valerian, Marsh Valerian, Pacific Valerian, *Fr.* Valériane de Sitka

PARTS USED: Root, rhizomes

CHARACTERISTICS: Spicy, bitter, warm

SYSTEMS AFFECTED: Liver, heart, nervous system

ACTIONS: Sedative, hypnotic, nervine, antispasmodic, carminative, stimulant, anodyne, hypotensive

RANGE: *V. officinalis* introduced in the Yukon, British Columbia, Manitoba to Newfoundland; *V. sitchensis* native to the Yukon, Northwest Territories, British Columbia, Alberta

Valerian's genus comprises about 150 species, the most widely used in herbology being the Garden Valerian (*V. officinalis*), which is native to Europe and Asia but is now present throughout most of Canada and has escaped to the wild. *V. sitchensis* is a native to Western Canada and considered to have stronger medicinal activity than the European variety. Attaining a height of 70 cm. up to 1 metre, it is smaller than Common Valerian, but is often one of the most abundant in the moist subalpine meadows of Western Canada. The flowers, which can be pink or white and fragrant, grow atop a usually smooth stem in two or more clusters or cymes. There are 2–4 pairs of compound opposite leaves with 1–4 pairs of lobes below a terminal leaflet. The plant sends out runners, spreading rather quickly, and the roots give off a rather fetid odour, somewhat like smelly socks. The root is more potent if kept from flowering and should be at least 2 years old; dig them up after the leaves have died down in the fall. Tincture and infusions are best made from the fresh root, but they may also be dried for later use.

MEDICINAL USES:

Insomnia, hypertension, menstrual cramps, eczema

- Eases pain and promotes sleep, helps with restless leg syndrome, anxiety, tension, and over-strained nerves. Should be used over a period of several weeks to be more effective.
- Studies show it may have a calming effect on people with obsessive-compulsive disorder and on hyperactive children. Often combined with Lemon Balm.
- Relieves menstrual cramps, intestinal colic, gas, muscle spasms, or cramps.
- Reduces blood pressure and calms agitated people. May be effective in the treatment of epilepsy.
- Externally an infusion can be used as a wash or compress to treat eczema and minor injuries or relieve muscle spasms.

OTHER USES: May be used to speed up bacterial activity in compost heaps as well as being a good fertilizer in gardens, attracting earthworms and adding phosphorus to the soil. Cats and rats are often attracted to it.

TINCTURE: 1–5 ml. (start with a smaller dose if it causes headache) taken an hour or two before bedtime.

COMBINATIONS:

May be mixed with Hops, St. John's Wort, and Skullcap for insomnia and anxiety.

CAUTION: No known side effects, although it's advisable to not exceed 3 months. Do not take with other sedatives or drive while taking.

VIOLET

Viola odorata
Viola adunca (Hooked Violet)

FAMILY: Violaceae

OTHER NAMES: Sweet Blue Violet, *Fr.* Violette odorante

PARTS USED: Aerial

CHARACTERISTICS: Sweet, mild but pleasantly bitter, cool

SYSTEMS AFFECTED: Lungs, stomach, liver, heart

ACTIONS: Demulcent, expectorant, astringent, alterative, febrifuge, antiseptic, vulnerary, anti-spasmodic, anodyne, antiscrofulous

RANGE: *V. odorata* introduced in British Columbia, Ontario, Quebec, Nova Scotia; *V. adunca* native across all of Canada; except Nunavut and Newfoundland and Labrador

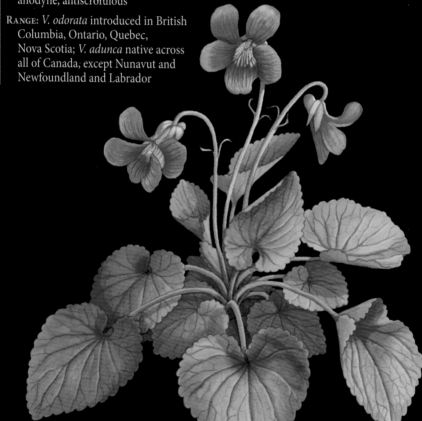

Violets are pretty little creeping perennials, some of which are native to Europe and others to North America, and which belong to a genus of over nine hundred species, all with similar medicinal uses:. Many foreign species have now naturalized throughout most of North America and are one of the first flowers to appear in the spring, traditionally symbolizing rebirth and bringing joy at the end of a long winter. Its leaves are heart-shaped, dark green, with scalloped edges, and grow in rosettes close to the ground. The fragrant flowers can be anywhere from deep purple to blue, pinkish, or even white. They are 5-petalled with a yellow beard in the centre and bloom from April to June. *V. adunca* is very similar to *V. odorata*, with a more elongated, hooked nectar spur on its flower. Oddly enough, the violet produces a second kind of flower later in the summer, growing colourless and hidden underground. Although they never see the light of day, they do produce viable seeds. If you pick only the leaves and flowers without disturbing the underground parts, they will continue to produce leaves all summer. Eat only the aerial parts, use fresh or dried, and store in glass away from heat and light.

MEDICINAL USES:

Dryness, inflammation, constipation, swollen glands, mastitis

- Very nourishing, rich in vitamins A and C and minerals, and may be added to Nettles for people with a dry constitution. Contains mucilage, which coats tissues and eases inflammation. Will soothe a sore throat or loosen mucous from the lungs when a cough is dry and unproductive.
- Laxative, the plant lubricates the intestines in cases of constipation.
- May be used in an eyewash to lubricate dry eyes.
- Chewed leaves can be applied to corns to soften skin or used as a poultice for hot, inflamed skin eruptions, or bug bites.
- May be used in oil for swollen glands or mastitis, massaged into the area. This is best complemented with an infusion taken internally. Acts as a lymphatic stimulant.
- Topically it is anti-inflammatory and can be used as a compress, infused oil, or salve to soothe dry or irritated skin, abrasions, insect bites, eczema, and hemorrhoids.
- Has a relaxing effect on the nervous system; contains methyl salicylate, a pain reliever, although in small quantity.
- Wonderful addition to salads.

INFUSION: 1 tbsp. dried or 2 tbsp. minced fresh herb steeped in 2 cups freshly boiled water for 10 minutes, or overnight. Strain and enjoy. May be combined with equal parts Dandelion leaf, Nettles, Red Clover, and Mint for a highly nutritious tea.

CAUTION: Underground parts should not be eaten as they can cause nausea and vomiting.

WESTERN MUGWORT

Artemisia ludoviciana

FAMILY: Asteraceae

OTHER NAMES: White Sagebrush, Silver Wormwood, Prairie Sage, Louisiana Wormwood, *Fr.* Armoise de l'Ouest

PARTS·USED: Leaves, flowering heads, roots

SYSTEMS AFFECTED: Liver, stomach, reproductive

CHARACTERISTICS: Bitter, acrid

ACTIONS: Astringent, antimicrobial, antioxidant, antifungal, anthelmintic, diaphoretic, emmenagogue, stimulant

RANGE: Native from British Columbia to Ontario, introduced in Quebec and New Brunswick

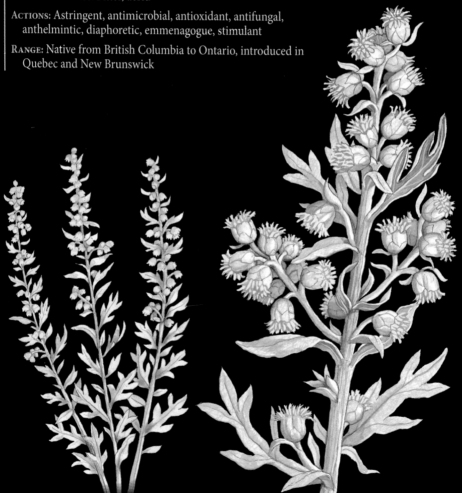

This aromatic perennial is one of many in this genus in North America that is often confused with others having similar common names and similar properties. This particular species is mostly a mountain dweller, grows about 90 cm. tall, and is found in stands of around 3 metres wide. The whole plant is light grey and covered with fine, downy hairs; its alternate leaves lance-shaped, sometimes deeply lobed, and may or may not have teeth. It is quite drought tolerant, and even becomes more aromatic when grown in poor, dry soil, its scent resembling that of Sagebrush. The small, yellow, tubular flowers grow on the upper branches from August to October, the tiny seeds ripening in late fall. Branches should be gathered when in flower, hung to dry, and stored in an airtight container out of the sunlight.

MEDICINAL USES:

Stomachache, gastric ulcers, delayed menstruation, diarrhea, pinworms, itchy skin, lung congestion

- Weak infusion is a common remedy used by Indigenous Peoples to relieve stomachache, diarrhea, and poor appetite, and to induce sweating when there is fever.
- Used externally for itching and rashes. Poultice of leaves relieves swellings, sores, boils, spider bites, and eczema. May be used as an underarm deodorant.
- Snuff made from the crushed, dry leaves used for sinus problems, headache, and nosebleeds.
- A handful of the herb added to a pot of boiling water can relieve sinus congestion, sore throat, colds, and bronchitis by inhaling the vapours through the mouth and nose. Add barley to the water to increase effectiveness.
- Liniment or infused oil rubbed on the joints helps ease the pain of rheumatism. Infused oil is applied to the skin for fungal infections.
- Effective against pinworm infections.
- Recent research, specifically with *A. ludoviciana ssp. mexicana,* has shown it may be effective against *H. pylori* related diseases (gastric ulcers) and could prove to be promising in the development of new treatments.

OTHER USES:
- Leaves may be placed in shoes to remove odour.
- Plant is burned to repel mosquitoes, as an incense, and for smudging and cleansing the air.

INFUSION: Standard cold infusion for stomach upset. Hot infusion as a diaphoretic to induce sweating or relieve menstrual cramps. Drink 4–6 tbsp. up to 4 times a day.

TINCTURE: Dried herb 1:5, in 50% alcohol. Take 20–40 drops up to 3 times a day.

CAUTION: Avoid during pregnancy. May cause allergies in some people.

WESTERN WHITE CLEMATIS

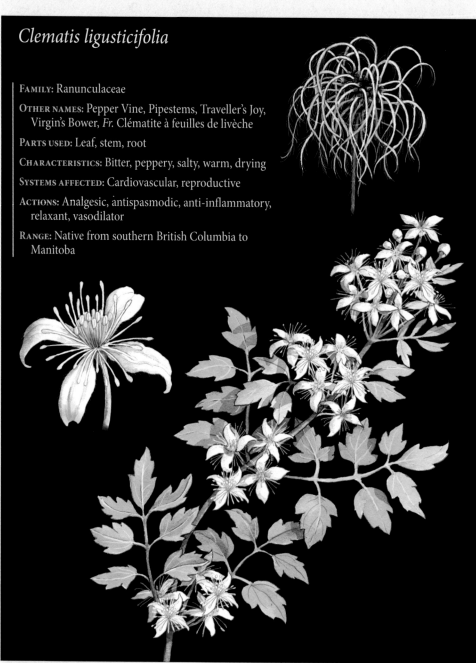

Clematis ligusticifolia

FAMILY: Ranunculaceae

OTHER NAMES: Pepper Vine, Pipestems, Traveller's Joy, Virgin's Bower, *Fr.* Clématite à feuilles de livèche

PARTS USED: Leaf, stem, root

CHARACTERISTICS: Bitter, peppery, salty, warm, drying

SYSTEMS AFFECTED: Cardiovascular, reproductive

ACTIONS: Analgesic, antispasmodic, anti-inflammatory, relaxant, vasodilator

RANGE: Native from southern British Columbia to Manitoba

This woody or semi-woody perennial is a vine that climbs over trees, shrubs, poles, or along the ground, often reaching a length of 6 metres or more. Preferring moist soil and wetlands, it grows mostly in semi-shade or woodlands. Like other members of the Buttercup genus, it contains compounds that can irritate the skin and mucous membranes; however, this species is not as toxic and is considered safe if used in small quantities. The leaves are opposite, pinnately compound with 5–7 leaflets that are irregularly lobed and coarsely toothed. From June to September it is covered with clusters of creamy white, fragrant blossoms that are replaced by feathery seed heads early in the fall. Flowers have 4 white sepals, no petals, and a creamy white-to-yellow centre of 25–50 stamens. The plant has more relaxant properties when leaves are picked before flowering. Use fresh or dry for later use.

MEDICINAL USES:

Migraines, uterine cramps, anxiety, sores, arthritis, bruises, sore throat

- Decoction of roots or snuff made from dried leaves dilates blood vessels to the brain, reducing severity of migraines and headaches if used as soon as symptoms appear.
- A poultice made from foliage is used to treat wounds, sores, burns, bruises, swellings, arthritic joints, muscle aches, and skin problems.
- The white of the bark is traditionally used by Indigenous Peoples to reduce fevers. Leaves and twigs are chewed to treat sore throats and colds. A decoction of the roots is taken for stomach aches.
- Relaxant, calms anxiety, relieves pain, and eases uterine cramps. Stalks and roots were once used as a contraceptive.
- Increases blood flow, warming, helps remove blood stagnation.

OTHER USES:
- Stems can be used to make string and bags.
- Roots are used in shampoos.
- Seed floss can be stuffed into shoes for insulation or used as tinder to start fires.

TINCTURE: Fresh plant 1:2, recently dried 1:5, in 50% alcohol. Take 10–40 drops up to 3 times a day.

INFUSION: Standard, 4–12 tbsp. up to twice a day.

CAUTION: Genus contains species that are toxic; use with caution. May cause burning of the mucous membranes or contact dermatitis. Avoid during pregnancy or breastfeeding or if using migraine medication. Use only in small amounts and avoid prolonged use.

WESTERN WILD GINGER

Asarum caudatum (Western)
A. canadense (Canadian)

FAMILY: Aristolochiaceae

OTHER NAMES: *A. caudatum*: British Columbia Wild Ginger, Long-tailed Wild Ginger, *Fr.* Asaret caudé; *A. canadense*: Canada Wild Ginger, Snakeroot, Colic Root, *Fr.* Asaret du Canada

PARTS USED: Rhizomes, leaves

SYSTEMS AFFECTED: Digestive, reproductive, cardiovascular

CHARACTERISTICS: Pungent, aromatic, warming

ACTIONS: Anthelmintic, analgesic, antirheumatic, carminative, diaphoretic, diuretic, laxative, stimulant, tonic

RANGE: *A. caudatum* native to British Columbia; *A. canadense* native to Manitoba, Ontario, Quebec, New Brunswick

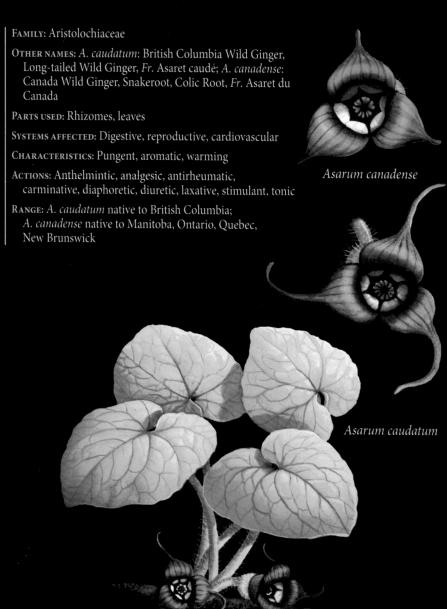

Asarum canadense

Asarum caudatum

This evergreen perennial is not a relative of culinary Ginger (*Zingiber officinale*), but its roots are occasionally used as a spice, exuding a mild ginger-like odour when crushed. A low-growing woodland plant about 15–25 cm. tall, it prefers shady, moist, acidic soils. The leaves grow in opposite pairs and are heart-shaped with a deep cleft at the base, the underside and stems covered in fine, white hairs. In the spring each plant produces a single, hairy, cup-shaped flower nestled beneath the carpet of leaves. They can be reddish, brownish-purple, or rust-coloured and have 3 triangular "petals" which are actually sepals; on the Western variety the tips are more elongated. Rhizomes grow close to the surface and are best harvested in early spring and fall, being careful not to unearth more than is needed. Dry for later use.

MEDICINAL USES:

Indigestion, cramping, dysmenorrhea, amenorrhea, colds, sore throat

- This plant, particularly leaves, stems and flowers, contains aristolochic acid, which can be toxic if taken in large quantities or over long periods of time. A decoction of the roots has been used by Indigenous Peoples for many years to ease intestinal cramps and digestive problems, to stimulate the appetite, or for colds, flus, and sore throat. Contains antibiotic substances which may be useful against certain bacteria and fungi, but more research is needed. Use with caution.
- Brings on delayed menstruation and relieves period cramps. Used by some Indigenous Peoples as a contraceptive by boiling the root for a long period of time and sipping the decoction.
- Decoction used externally for headaches, joint pain. Fresh warmed leaves may be applied to wounds, boils, skin infections and toothaches. Used in compounds for fractures.
- Strengthens the effect of other herbs when used in formulas.

OTHER USES:
- Dried root burned as incense.
- Repels insects.
- Decoction may be used as an herbicide.

DECOCTION: Standard decoction, sip 6–8 tbsp. up to 3 times a day.

TINCTURE: Fresh root 1:2, dried 1:5 in 60% alcohol. Take 20–40 drops in hot water.

CAUTION: Contains aristolochic acid, a toxin that can cause kidney damage and cancer. Do not use if pregnant or breastfeeding. Avoid in inflammatory conditions. Handling may cause dermatitis in some people. Use only in small quantities and over a short period of time.

WHITE HOREHOUND

Marrubium vulgare

FAMILY: Lamiaceae or Labiatae

OTHER NAMES: Common Horehound, *Fr.* Marrube blanc

PARTS USED: Aerial

SYSTEMS AFFECTED: Digestive, Respiratory, Cardiovascular

CHARACTERISTICS: Bitter, pungent

ACTIONS: Antibacterial, antispasmodic, antioxidant, anti-inflammatory, analgesic, cholagogue, diaphoretic, digestive, diuretic, emmenagogue, expectorant, hepatic, hypoglycemic, stimulant, tonic

RANGE: Introduced in southern British Columbia, Saskatchewan, Ontario, Quebec, Nova Scotia

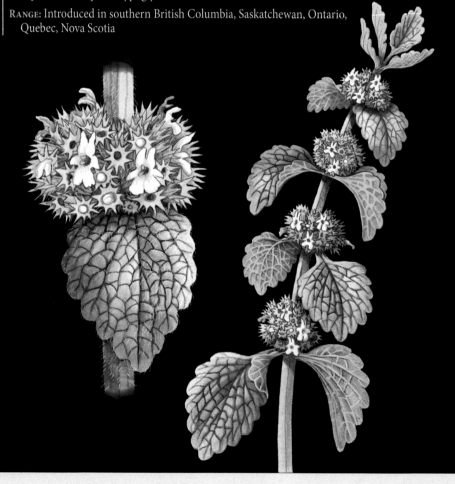

This plant from the mint family is a native of Europe, Northern Africa, and western Asia that has become naturalized in North America and is cultivated more and more due to its vast potential for medicinal use. Its Latin name *Marrubium* stems from the Hebrew marrob meaning "bitter juice," which describes its taste and function as a digestive herb, but it is better known for its effectiveness as a cough remedy. Its branched stems, which can reach from 30–90 cm. tall, are square and hairy, the downy, wrinkled leaves round or ovate with rounded teeth, arranged in opposite pairs along the stems. The small, white, tubular flowers, which come out in the spring, are arranged in axillary whorls around the stem. As they mature, the calyces' spiny teeth once dried will cling to passersby to disperse their seeds. Found along roadsides and in fields, the plants can be harvested in spring as they start flowering, and may be used fresh for tincturing or dried for later use in teas.

MEDICINAL USES:

Coughs and other upper respiratory problems, fever, amenorrhea, hypertension, indigestion, wounds

- Effective expectorant, commonly used in cough medicines for hoarseness, asthma, bronchitis, and other respiratory ailments. Loosens phlegm and breaks up congestion, tones the mucous membranes. A hot infusion will promote sweating when there is fever.
- Normalizes heart rhythm, decreases systolic blood pressure, mild cardiotonic.
- Cool infusion or tincture helps ease indigestion, flatulence, loss of appetite. Gastroprotective, helps ulcers, jaundice.
- Has antimicrobial activity against fungi, herpes simplex virus, and some parasites. Essential oil is a natural insecticide.
- Externally, it is used to heal wounds, skin damage, and ulcers.
- Traditional use by some Indigenous Peoples (with equal portion of Plantain) for rattlesnake bite.
- Ongoing research suggests it could have anti-cancer properties and effectiveness in treating diabetes mellitus, but more study is needed.

COUGH SYRUP: Bring 2 tbsp. of dried herb and 1 cup water to a boil, and simmer for 30 minutes covered. Strain, cool slightly, and add 1 cup unpasteurized honey. Add lime or lemon juice and ½ cup brandy if desired.

COLD INFUSION: Diuretic. Place 2 tbsp. dried herb into a cheesecloth bag and suspend in 4 cups of cold water. Leave overnight, then remove bag, squeezing out all the liquid. Take 4–8 tbsp. up to 4 times a day.

WARM INFUSION: Diaphoretic. Standard, 4–8 tbsp. up to 4 times a day.

TINCTURE: Fresh 1:2, dried 1:5 in 50% alcohol. Take 30–90 drops, 4 times a day.

CAUTION: Avoid if pregnant or nursing. May cause diarrhea in large doses.

WILD LICORICE

Glycyrrhiza lepidota

FAMILY: Fabaceae or Leguminosae

OTHER NAMES: American Licorice, *Fr.* Réglisse sauvage

PARTS USED: Root, leaves

SYSTEMS AFFECTED: Respiratory, digestive

CHARACTERISTICS: Sweet, moist, cooling

ACTIONS: Antibacterial, antimicrobial, antioxidant, antifungal, anti-inflammatory, demulcent, expectorant, emollient, respiratory and kidney stimulant

RANGE: Native from southeast British Columbia to western Ontario

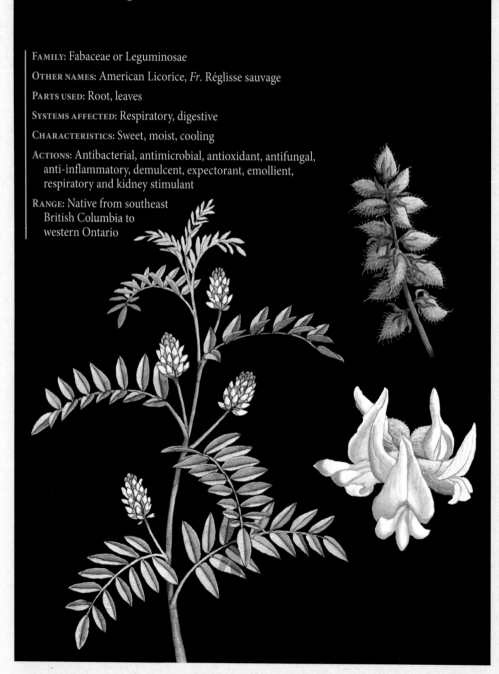

The European variety of Licorice (*G. glabra*) has a very long history of use around the world and has been cultivated both as a medicine and a flavouring for centuries. The American wild variety is perhaps less well-known, but is widely used by Indigenous Peoples across North America for much the same purposes. A perennial from the pea family, it grows up to around 1 metre, its erect stem producing alternate compound leaves composed of up to 21 oblong toothless leaflets which often fold up when young. The flowers grow in mid to late summer from the leaf axils in spiky clusters and range from white to cream or pale yellow in colour. They are replaced by a green pod of about 1.3 cm. long which is covered in hooked bristles and turns brown as it matures, often sticking to animal fur. Its woody roots or horizontal rhizomes, which are primarily used for medicines, taste like Licorice and are sweet due to the presence of glycyrrhizin, a substance fifty times sweeter than sugar. Plant should be at least 3 or 4 years old before harvesting. Dig up root in the fall, split lengthwise and dry for later use.

MEDICINAL USES:

Coughs and upper respiratory problems, fever, stomachache, toothache, sores

- Peeled, dry root is used in decoction as an effective expectorant, commonly used for coughs and other inflammatory upper respiratory infections, bronchial asthma, sore throat, and fevers in children. Added to medicines and syrups to sweeten the taste.
- Sipping an infusion will speed up delivery of the placenta in childbirth.
- Good remedy for stomachaches and diarrhea.
- Chewing the dried root is effective in easing toothache pain or sore throat. When saliva is swallowed after chewing, it helps strengthen the voice of singers.
- Externally, it can be used as a wash or poultice for swellings, and the mashed leaves may be applied to sores on both humans and animals.
- Taking 2 cups of infusion per day for 1 week lessens painful menstrual cramps.
- Ongoing research suggests the plant may inhibit growth of HIV-infected white blood cells.

OTHER USES:
- Roots may be eaten raw, cooked, or slow-roasted.
- Roots chewed by Indigenous Peoples as a tooth cleaner, or to cool the body in sweat lodges or Sun Dance ceremonies.
- Tender spring shoots can be eaten raw in the spring.
- Powdered roots are used as a sweetener.

DECOCTION: Strong decoction, 2–6 tbsp. up to 3 times a day.

COMBINATIONS:

Strengthens the effect of other herbs. Works well with Mullein and Horehound for coughs; Echinacea, Ginseng, Hawthorn for strengthening the immune system, heart, adrenals and nervous system.

CAUTION: Avoid if pregnant or nursing. May increase blood pressure; increased risk of edema, headaches, sluggishness if taken in large quantities.

YARROW

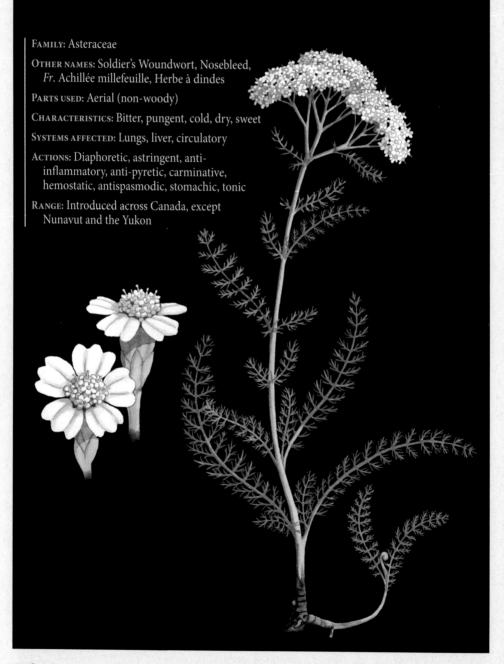

Achillea millefolium

FAMILY: Asteraceae

OTHER NAMES: Soldier's Woundwort, Nosebleed, *Fr.* Achillée millefeuille, Herbe à dindes

PARTS USED: Aerial (non-woody)

CHARACTERISTICS: Bitter, pungent, cold, dry, sweet

SYSTEMS AFFECTED: Lungs, liver, circulatory

ACTIONS: Diaphoretic, astringent, anti-inflammatory, anti-pyretic, carminative, hemostatic, antispasmodic, stomachic, tonic

RANGE: Introduced across Canada, except Nunavut and the Yukon

This common perennial weed found throughout North America has been popular as a medicinal herb for centuries. It gets its name from the Greek myth of Achilles, who was invulnerable to arrows except on his heel, and it was traditionally used to stop the bleeding of soldier's wounds on battlefields. It grows 20–90 cm. tall, with stems branching near the top and alternate, highly segmented, feathery leaves. At the top of the stalk are clusters of tiny white or pink daisy-like flowers with 5 petals which bloom throughout the summer and fall. It grows in fields and on roadsides but is more potent if found in stony, sandy soils, and should be harvested early in the summer. Avoid using the woody stalks and mature leaves. Hang to dry.

MEDICINAL USES:

Wounds, fever, colds and flu, poor digestion, urinary tract infections, menstrual cramps, hemorrhoids

- Has been used as a wound remedy since Roman times, being especially good for deep wounds that bleed profusely. It will stop hemorrhaging and at the same time break up congealed blood or bruises. May be used internally or externally as a poultice. Indigenous Peoples use it in teas or pound the plant into a pulp for sprains, bruises, and wounds.
- Relieves fever by causing sweating; good for colds and flu, especially in children. May be used along with Peppermint and Elderflower.
- Used for chronic urinary tract infections, incontinence and leukorrhea.
- Bitter, stimulates stomach acids to aid digestion of fats and proteins, helps heartburn. Soothes mild diarrhea and dysentery.
- Helps ease menstrual cramps and normalizes irregular periods.
- Tones the blood vessels, relieves bleeding hemorrhoids and varicose veins as well as internal bleeding and ulcers. Also tones the mucous membranes of the digestive tract; particularly useful for dysentery, colitis, and leaky gut.
- May be used in a sitz bath to help with uterine fibroids, varicose veins, hemorrhoids, leukorrhea, rashes, or eczema.
- Anti-inflammatory, eases pain of osteoarthritis.
- Good for countering the side-effects from radiation therapy and hot flashes.

INFUSION: 1–2 tsp. dried herb in 1 cup boiling water, infuse 10–15 minutes. Drink hot 3 times a day. For fevers drink hourly.

TINCTURES: 2–4 ml. 3 times a day.

SITZ BATH: ½ cup whole cut herb steeped in cold water overnight. Bring to boil, strain and add to sitz bath water.

CAUTION: Avoid using over a long period of time. Not advised during pregnancy.

YELLOW DOCK

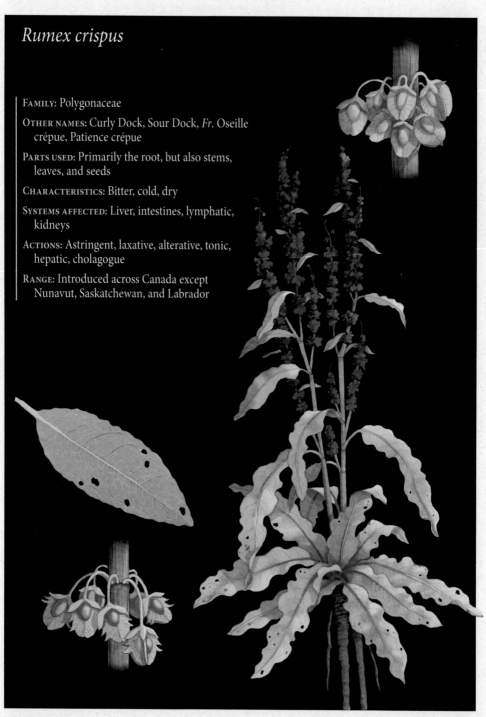

Rumex crispus

FAMILY: Polygonaceae

OTHER NAMES: Curly Dock, Sour Dock, *Fr.* Oseille crépue, Patience crépue

PARTS USED: Primarily the root, but also stems, leaves, and seeds

CHARACTERISTICS: Bitter, cold, dry

SYSTEMS AFFECTED: Liver, intestines, lymphatic, kidneys

ACTIONS: Astringent, laxative, alterative, tonic, hepatic, cholagogue

RANGE: Introduced across Canada except Nunavut, Saskatchewan, and Labrador

This common perennial weed is native to Europe and Africa but is now found throughout most of North America. As its names imply, it has broad, wavy, crinkled leaves, crisp around the edges, with a long tap root that's usually not forked, and yellow inside with thick rusty brown bark. Its close relative, *Rumex obtusifolius*, or Bitter Dock, has similar properties and is distinguished by its wider, flat leaves and tiny spikes on its seedpods. Both are tenacious weeds, often despised by gardeners, as each root must be dug out in its entirety since even the smallest piece left in the ground will produce another plant. The stem grows up to 90 cm. high, with green flower spikes branching off at intervals, producing an abundance of rust-coloured seed spikes in late summer and fall. The roots should be dug up in late summer or early fall; clean well and split lengthwise before drying.

MEDICINAL USES:

Liver sluggishness, constipation, skin irritations, anemia, throat and gum inflammation, eczema, arthritis

- Digestive tonic that acts specifically on the liver, gallbladder, and kidneys, promoting bile production, cleansing, assisting digestion of fats and proteins. This in turn improves conditions related to sluggish liver, including acne, psoriasis, headaches, constipation, arthritis, and long-term chronic diseases of the intestinal tract. Good for chronic constipation as it gently stimulates peristalsis and increases mucous production in the colon. Add Fennel or cumin seed if desired. Avoid long-term use.
- Contains many nutrients, but particularly rich in iron. Cleanses and nourishes the blood and is helpful in formulas as a remedy for anemia. Strengthens capillaries, helps hemorrhoids, varicose veins, internal bleeding.
- Decoction of the boiled stems or roots can be used in an ointment made with beeswax and olive oil to relieve itching, eczema, psoriasis, or other irritations. The decoction also works topically as an antiseptic and astringent to treat wounds, swellings, burns, hemorrhoids, and insect bites. Young shoots when rubbed on the skin will help soothe nettle stings. The mashed root pulp is used as a poultice by Indigenous Peoples for swellings and sores.
- Young shoots are very nutritious and can be boiled and eaten. Good for rheumatism.
- Commonly used for inflammations of the nasal passages, throat, and gums as well as coughs and bronchitis.

DECOCTION: 1 tsp. dried root in 1 cup water. Decoct 10–15 minutes, steep another 30 minutes. Take ½ cup 2–3 times a day.

SYRUP: For anemia or blood deficiency, add Nettles, Peony root, Red Clover, and molasses to decoction. Take 1 cup 3 times a day for no more than 3 months.

TINCTURE: Fresh 1:2, dried 1:5, in 50% alcohol. Take 1–2 ml. 3 times a day.

CAUTION: Should not be taken in combination with other diuretics, Lasix, or other drugs treating congestive heart failure or edema, as it can cause potassium depletion. Do not consume in large quantities or over a long period of time.

YELLOW GENTIAN

Gentiana lutea
G. sceptrum (King's Sceptre Gentian)

FAMILY: Gentianaceae

OTHER NAMES: Bitterroot, Gall Weed, *Fr.* Gentiane Jaune

PARTS USED: Root, rhizomes

SYSTEMS AFFECTED: Stomach, liver, gallbladder, central nervous system

CHARACTERISTICS: Bitter, cool

ACTIONS: Anthelmintic, anti-inflammatory, antiseptic, cholagogue, tonic, gastric stimulant, stomachic

RANGE: *G. lutea* introduced in Alberta; *G. sceptrum* native to British Columbia

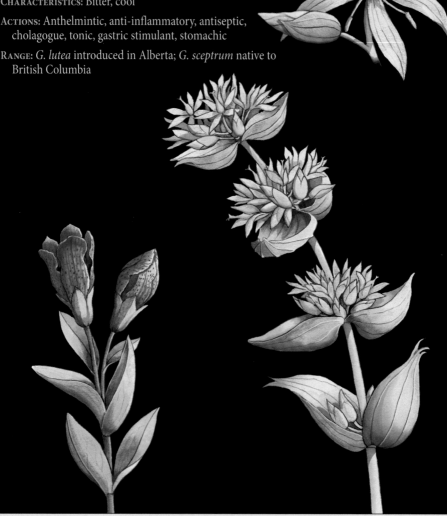

One of the strongest bitter herb tonics available, Yellow Gentian is well known in herbal medicine for treating digestive problems. A native of Europe, Africa, and Asia, it was used by the ancient Egyptians, Romans, and Greeks for centuries. Across Canada it's often cultivated but has only been found growing wild in a few locations in Alberta. It is most often in alpine meadows, moist grasslands, and pastures, and can reach a height of about a metre. Its large oval or lance-shaped basal leaves have deep ribbed veins, and the flower stalk emerges in summer with whorled clusters of star-shaped blooms growing from the axils of the upper leaves. The large taproot can be at least 30 cm. long and is often 5 cm. thick. Harvest in the fall after several years of growth but preferably before flowering, which takes about three years. Dry for later use. King's Sceptre Gentian is not known for its medicinal properties, but its blue flower may be used in dyes and soaps.

MEDICINAL USES:

Digestive problems, constipation, worms, liver congestion and jaundice, upper respiratory tract infections, food allergies and cravings, loss of appetite, exhaustion

- This root is so bitter it can be detected even in a dilution of 1:50,000; however, this allows it to tone the digestive system better than any other herb, stimulating the mouth and digestive tract to release more enzymes. Used especially for post-viral syndrome, states of exhaustion from chronic disease, and weakness of the digestive system causing lack of appetite, food intolerances, bloating, and sluggishness. It stimulates the liver, gallbladder, and pancreas.
- Loosens blocked mucous from sinuses and bronchi, reduces inflammation in the nose and throat.
- Antibacterial and antimicrobial actions improve circulation and cardiovascular system, speeding up healing of wounds and reducing pain.
- Expels worms.
- Low doses stimulate the nerves; higher doses settle the nerves and ease anxiety.

TINCTURE: Dried 1:2 in 50% alcohol, 6–12 drops 3–5 minutes before eating. May be taken diluted in water if it is found to be too strong, however it is important to taste the bitterness in order for the medicine to work, so avoid diluting too much.

COMBINATIONS:

Mix 2 parts Gentian with 1 part Ginger root to improve taste and add warmth. May be combined with Primrose flowers, Sorrel, Elder flowers, and Vervain to help sinusitis.

CAUTION: Do not exceed recommended dose. Use only dried root, as fresh may cause nausea. Avoid if you have stomach ulcers, gallstones, or blocked bile ducts, excessive stomach acid, and heartburn. Not recommended during pregnancy.

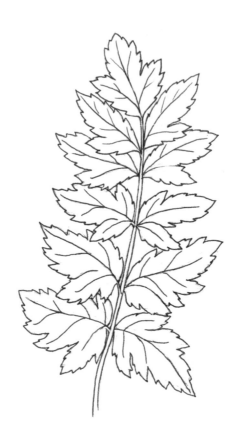

POISONOUS PLANTS

This section deals with those plants we must be extra careful to avoid, since it is very easy when wildcrafting to mistake one plant for another and sometimes this can have dire consequences. I focussed on plants that are primarily toxic to handle, although many of them are also poisonous when ingested. Garden plants and the ones already mentioned have not been included.

Apiaceae Family

Plants in this family are tricky to identify and include edible plants like Carrots, Parsnip, Parsley, Fennel, and Dill; however, there are many others that can be extremely toxic although they may closely resemble their edible relatives. Identification by the flowers, which are usually white and in clusters arranged in umbels or umbrella-like formations, is particularly confusing. These plants contain chemicals in the sap which cause phytophotosensitivity, or extreme sensitivity to sunlight if the skin comes in contact with them. A good rule is: if you're not 100% sure what it is, leave it alone!

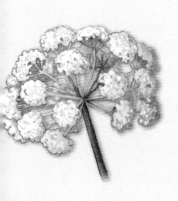

| TREATMENT |

If you accidentally touch any of these plants, immediately keep the skin away from sunlight and wash the area with cool running water. Avoid rubbing or using hot water as this will open the pores and allow the poison to go deeper. Do not touch other areas of the body, particularly the eyes. Use a mild soap to remove any remaining residue. If there is soreness, cover area with a cool, damp cloth. If there are open sores or blistering, apply an antibiotic cream and sterile bandage, changing at least twice a day. When a large area is affected, see a doctor.

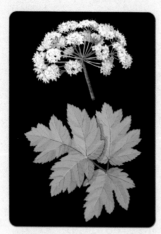

COW PARSNIP
Heracleum maximum (lanatum)

- Native, the Yukon to Newfoundland.
- Sap contains furanocoumarins, which will cause photo dermatitis; handle with gloves and use extreme caution when foraging or trimming. When exposed to sun, may cause rashes that could persist for months.
- Grows up to 3 metres tall. Flower umbels may be up to 20 cm. in diameter. Leaves are up to 60 cm. wide and hairy, and are divided into 3 deeply lobed leaflets. Lobes are more rounded than those of Giant Hogweed. Stem has some purple areas and deep ridges.
- Young leaves and flower pods may be eaten cooked, and seeds when dry and brown can be used as a spice. Plant is no longer toxic when dried or cooked. It is extremely important to properly identify before consuming, as it is similar to other poisonous plants.

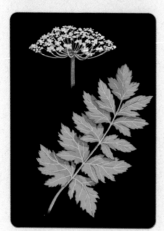

WILD PARSNIP
Pastinaca sativa

- Introduced, the Yukon to Newfoundland, invasive.
- Sap contains furanocoumarins, which will cause photo dermatitis. Handle only with gloves.
- In the first year it grows a rosette of basal leaves, the second year the tall flower stalk appears, and then the plant dies.
- Flowers grow in yellowish-green umbels. Grows up to 1.5 metres tall; its single smooth stem is deeply grooved with few hairs. Leaves are compound, its toothed leaflets arranged in pairs with a single leaf at the tip. Seeds are brown and flat.

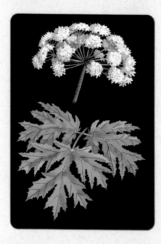

GIANT HOGWEED
Heracleum mantegazzianum

- Introduced, British Columbia, Ontario to Newfoundland, invasive.
- Sap contains furanocoumarins, which will cause severe photo dermatitis; avoid contact.
- Mature plant can reach 5 metres in height. Hollow stem is green with reddish-purple blotches or be entirely purple, with a rough texture and stiff hairs. The compound leaves can be up to 1.5 metres long, are shiny and deeply divided into lobed leaflets with coarse, serrated edges. White umbels can be up to 60 cm. in diameter.

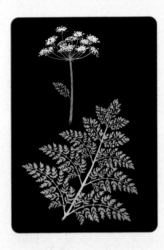

POISON HEMLOCK
Conium maculatum

- Introduced, British Columbia to Saskatchewan, Ontario to Nova Scotia, invasive.
- Biennial; up to 3 metres tall in second year. Branching stem is hollow, red or purple spotted, smooth, and hairless. Leaves are compound with leaflets growing in pairs from opposite sides of leaf stalk, finely divided and feathery, much like Queen Anne's Lace or Parsley. They give off a strong musty odour when crushed. Flowers grow in rounded clusters 5–7.5 cm. in diameter.
- Contains the alkaloid coniine. All parts of the plant are poisonous and even remain toxic for up to three years after dying off. Eating the plant is the most dangerous, but the poisons can also affect the skin and respiratory system. Symptoms include dizziness, trembling, paralysis, and eventually death due to respiratory failure. Quick treatment can reverse the harm, but an immediate response is necessary.

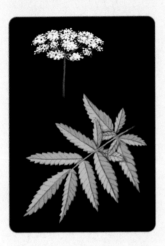

WATER HEMLOCK
Cicuta maculata (Spotted)
Cicuta douglasii (Western)

- *Cicuta maculata* is native across Canada except Newfoundland and Labrador. *Cicuta douglasii* is native to the Yukon, British Columbia, Alberta.
- Contains cicutoxin, which is present in all parts of the plant. It is one of the deadliest plants in North America. A piece of the root the size of a walnut is enough to kill a cow.
- Perennial, grows up to 2 metres tall, typically in wetlands and along streams.
- Stem is smooth, mostly hairless and hollow, sometimes branching and usually with purple streaks or stripes. Leaves are two or three times pinnate with a single leaf at the top, have lance-shaped, sharply toothed leaflets with veins that terminate in notches, not at the tips. Flowers are white, growing in compound umbels about 15 cm. across.

Other Species to Avoid

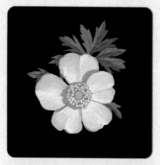

BUTTERCUP (most species)
Ranunculus

- Native across all of Canada.
- Contains protoanemonin, an acrid, toxic oil which can cause itching and burning of the skin and irritate the eyes, and if chewed can create blisters in the mouth and on the face. If swallowed they can cause severe gastrointestinal irritation, spasms, and paralysis.
- Family consists of several hundred species with varying levels of the toxic compound, including popular garden plants like *Clematis*, *Helleborus*, *Pulsatilla* and *Anemone*. They have alternate, palmately veined leaves that may be entire, lobed, or finely divided. Flowers are usually yellow, but may be any colour, with 5 petals; can grow singly or in loose clusters.

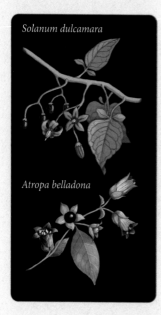

Solanum dulcamara

Atropa belladona

NIGHTSHADE
Solanum dulcamara (Bittersweet Nightshade)

Atropa belladonna (Deadly Nightshade)

- *Solanum dulcamara* was introduced in British Columbia, Saskatchewan, and Ontario to Newfoundland. *Atropa belladonna* was introduced in southern British Columbia (rare).
- *S. dulcamara* is a perennial vine or shrub with purple, star-shaped flowers with a prominent yellow centre growing in clusters along the vine. Berries are egg-shaped and green when unripe, changing to bright red as they ripen. Leaves are dark green, often with one or two lobes near the base, and emit an unpleasant smell when crushed. The entire plant contains solanine, a toxin found in green potatoes and other nightshades, and dulcamarine, similar to the toxin found in Deadly Nightshade. Although not as toxic as Deadly Nightshade, the leaves, green berries, and even ripe berries can be poisonous if ingested.
- *A. belladonna* is a perennial which contains atropine, along with other toxic alkaloids, in all parts of the plant, particularly in the sweet, black berries which can be confused with blueberries or black currants. Can cause increased heart rate, dilated pupils, hallucinations, vomiting, respiratory failure, and death. It grows as a shrub of up to 1.5 metres with single, greenish-purple star-shaped bell flowers growing from the leaf axils. Leaves are dark green, alternate, smooth, and oval. Contact a physician immediately if poisoning is suspected.

POISON OAK
Toxicodendron diversilobum (Western Poison Oak)

POISON IVY
Toxicodendron radicans (Western Poison Ivy)

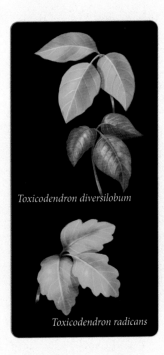

Toxicodendron diversilobum

Toxicodendron radicans

- *Toxicodendron diversilobum* is native to British Columbia. *Toxicodendron radicans* is native from the Yukon to Nova Scotia, introduced to Newfoundland.
- Poison Oak grows as a shrub, ground vine, or woody vine that wraps around trees for up to 30 metres; Western Poison Ivy grows only as a ground vine. Leaves vary in colour, from green with tinges of red in the spring to shiny green to red in the fall. Each leaf consists of three leaflets from 2.5–15 cm. long. Poison Oak leaves resemble Oak leaves with irregular, rounded lobes, whereas Poison Ivy has leaflets that may or may not be lobed and have pointed tips. Tiny flowers are greenish-white, growing in clusters on a stem, and the fruit are whitish glossy berries with ridges; they become dry with a papery shell when ripe.
- Contains the oil urushiol, which can be transferred to the skin from direct contact or contact with objects, clothing, or other people or animals that have touched the plant. It can remain for long periods of time and can only be degraded by washing thoroughly with soap and water; however, it can even remain in the water or washing machine and be transferred to other clothing. Causes severe contact dermatitis, itching, swelling, and blisters. Inhalation of smoke from burning plants can cause respiratory tract inflammation that may require hospitalization.
- If you've been exposed, wash skin thoroughly with soap and water as soon as possible, trying not to spread the oil to other areas. Take an oral antihistamine to reduce itching, apply calamine lotion, or take oatmeal baths or compresses to soothe irritation. Avoid scratching or touching the area. Seek medical advice if large areas have been affected.

SPURGE-LAUREL
Daphne laureola

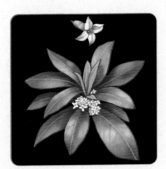

- Introduced in British Columbia; invasive.
- Evergreen shrub that grows to a height of up to 1.3 metres. Dark green leaves are glossy, thick, oval-shaped, and grow in a spiral pattern around the top of the stem. Twigs have a strong smell when cut. Small, fragrant flowers are light green with orange stamens and grow in clusters at the base of the leaves, followed by black berries in the early summer.
- Leaves, berries, and sap contain irritating toxins that cause severe skin irritation and blistering if touched, or burning of the mouth and lips and swelling of the tongue, difficulty swallowing, nausea, and diarrhea if berries are ingested. Flush with water if touched, and apply antihistamine cream to reduce irritation. Contact a physician immediately if ingested.

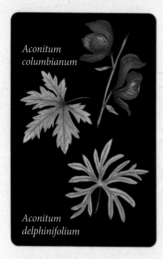

Aconitum columbianum

Aconitum delphinifolium

MONKSHOOD

Aconitum columbianum (Columbian Monkshood)

Aconitum delphinifolium (Mountain Monkshood)

- *Aconitum columbianum* is native to British Columbia. *Aconitum delphinifolium* is native to the Yukon, Northwest Territories, British Columbia, Alberta.
- Herbaceous perennial identified by the sepal or outer part of the flower that resembles a hood. They typically grow vertically on upright stems in racemes or groups and vary in colour from blue to white. Alternate leaves are usually 5-lobed and deeply cleft. Height of *A. columbianum* can be up to 2 metres, but *A. delphinifolium* is much smaller at 50 cm.
- All parts are poisonous, most severely from ingesting, but toxins can also be absorbed through the skin. Contains the alkaloid aconitine, which mainly affects the heart but can also cause nausea, chest pain, diarrhea, dizziness, shortness of breath. Seek medical help immediately.

GLOSSARY

Abortifacient A substance that brings on an abortion.

Adaptogen Herbs that work on the immune and neuro-endocrine systems, increasing the body's resistance and adaptability to stress while balancing the overall physiology without being toxic, even with long-term use. Tonic, antioxidant, and anti-inflammatory, not specific to any organ but help regulate organ and system function in general and maintain homeostasis.

Adjuvant A substance that aids the action of a medicinal agent or medical treatment.

Alterative A medicine that favourably alters the course of an ailment and gradually restores health.

Amenorrhea Absence of menstruation, usually due to either stress, weight gain or loss, excessive exercise, cysts or tumours, hormonal imbalance, pregnancy or lactation. May be erratic, occurring for short periods of time.

Analeptic An agent that has a restorative or stimulating effect, as on the central nervous system; may act as an anticonvulsant.

Analgesic An agent that relieves pain.

Anaphrodisiac An agent that reduces one's capacity for sexual arousal.

Anodyne An agent that relieves pain or promotes comfort, usually externally.

Anthelmintic A substance that kills and expels intestinal parasitic worms.

Antibiotic An agent that inhibits the growth of or kills an organism, usually in reference to bacteria or micro-organisms.

Antifungal An agent that kills or stops the growth of fungi or yeast which can cause infections in the body.

Anti-inflammatory An agent that reduces redness, heat, and swelling of inflamed tissues.

Antilithic A substance that dissolves or reduces the size of kidney stones.

Antioxidant An agent that helps protect the body from damage by free radicals, a major cause of disease and aging.

Antipyretic An agent that prevents or reduces fever.

Antirheumatic A substance that is used in the treatment of arthritis.

Antiscorbutic A substance that prevents or cures scurvy.

Antitussive A substance that relieves coughs.

Aperient An agent that is mildly purgative or laxative.

Astringent Remedies that cause soft tissues to pucker or draw together, usually due to the presence of tannins. They are useful for reducing irritation and inflammation and create a barrier against infection in wounds and burns. They diminish secretions, check minor bleeding, and control diarrhea. Not recommended for long-term use.

Bitters Herbs having a bitter taste which stimulate digestive juices and bile production, and subsequently increase appetite. They may also stimulate peristalsis and help repair damage in the gastrointestinal wall.

Carminative Soothes the gut, easing pain and causing release of stomach or intestinal gas. This action is due to the presence of volatile oils, which have anti-inflammatory, antispasmodic, and antimicrobial effects on the lining of the intestines.

Catarrh A condition where the mucous membranes of the nose and breathing passages are inflamed, often chronically.

Cathartic A purgative or laxative causing evacuation of the bowels.

Cholagogue An agent that increases the flow of bile from the gallbladder, which in turn facilitates fat digestion and works as a natural laxative. Should not be used with toxic liver disorders, acute viral hepatitis, painful gallstones, or other acute liver problems.

Cystitis A urinary tract infection characterized by inflammation in the bladder, most commonly in women.

Decoction A herbal preparation of roots or woody plant material boiled in water.

Demulcent Herbs which tend to become slimy in water and work to form a barrier on irritated tissues, soothing inflammation of the mucous membranes. They reduce irritation all through the digestive tract, easing muscle spasms and sensitivity to gastric acids, as well as easing coughs, sore throats, and pain in the bladder and urinary systems.

Depurative An agent that has a purifying effect.

Diaphoretic An agent that usually works by relaxing the sweat glands and inducing a greater outward flow of blood, thereby increasing the amount of perspiration. This rids the body of offensive materials and aids the immune and endocrine systems.

Diffusive Having the effect of spreading every way by flowing and improving circulation of fluids.

Diuretic Agents that help the body get rid of excess fluids by increasing urine flow, helping with a wide range of disorders where too much fluid accumulates in the tissues (edema).

Dropsy An old-fashioned term for edema or lymph congestion.

Dysmenorrhea Painful menstruation with cramping, due to a variety of underlying causes.

Edema A buildup of fluids in the tissues causing swelling.

Emetic An agent that induces vomiting.

Emmenagogue An agent that regulates and stimulates normal menstruation, as well as having a toning effect on the female reproductive system.

Emollient Having the ability to soften and moisturize the skin.

Expectorant An agent that facilitates the expulsion of phlegm from the respiratory tract by irritating and stimulating the bronchioles to liquefy and move thick sputum upwards so it can be cleared more easily by coughing, or by relaxing and loosening thinner mucous as in a dry cough.

Febrifuge An agent that relieves fever.

Galactagogue An agent that promotes the flow of milk.

Hemostatic An agent that controls or stops bleeding.

Hepatic A remedy that supports the liver by toning, strengthening and in some cases detoxifying and increasing the flow of bile, which in turn affects the entire digestive system.

Hypertensive An agent that causes a rise in blood pressure.

Hypnotic Herbs that promote sleep and have a relaxing effect on the nervous system.

Hyperglycemia When there are high levels of glucose or blood sugar in the blood due to too little insulin or inability to use insulin properly. Typical in people with diabetes.

Hypoglycemia When the level of glucose or blood sugar drops to levels that are unhealthy, most common in people with diabetes.

Hypotensive An agent that reduces elevated blood pressure.

Infusion A herbal preparation made by soaking the herbs in hot or cold water to be drunk as a tea.

Leukorrhea Thick, white vaginal discharge.

Lymphatic The system in the body which consists of a network of delicate tubes or vessels that drain fluid (lymph) that has seeped from the blood vessels into the tissues and returns it to the bloodstream through the lymph nodes. Includes the tonsils, spleen, and thymus. An important part of the immune system.

Mastitis Inflammation of the breast tissue due to infection, mainly affecting breastfeeding women, that results in pain, swelling, and redness, and sometimes fever and chills.

Menorrhagia Excessive menstrual bleeding, in younger women usually as a result of fibroids, tumours, polyps, endometriosis, or blood-clotting problems, in older women typically caused by erratic hormones due to perimenopause.

Mucilaginous Containing a gel-like, slimy substance called mucilage which can be helpful to soothe inflammation.

Nervine An agent that has a beneficial effect on the nervous system. Depending on the plant, this can work as a tonic, which repairs damage to the nervous system in cases of trauma or stress; as a relaxant, which eases anxiety and relaxes the peripheral nerves, muscles, and organs of the body; or as a stimulant, which helps enhance vitality where the body is sluggish.

Neuroprotective An agent that protects nerve cells from damage or degeneration by pathogens in neurodegenerative diseases.

Pectoral Relating to the chest or thorax; between the neck and abdomen.

Peristalsis A series of wave-like involuntary contractions of the muscles that move food along the digestive tract.

Parturient A substance which aids in the birthing process.

Poultice A warm mass of plant material, or a cloth wrapped in plant material, which is applied to the skin to cause a medicinal action.

Purgative An agent that acts as a strong laxative, cleansing the bowel, often with cramping and pain.

Restorative An agent or medicine that is able to restore health, strength, and well-being.

Rubefacient Causes localized reddening of the skin.

Saponin A compound in some plants that has a foaming or soapy action when shaken with water. Effects the immune system by reducing inflammation, lowers blood lipids, and reduces the risk of cancer.

Scrofula Swellings of the lymph glands in the neck, commonly caused by tuberculosis.

Styptic A substance that slows or stops bleeding by contracting the blood vessels; astringent.

Stomachic An agent that aids the stomach and digestion.

Tincture A herbal medicine prepared by soaking plant material in alcohol, cider vinegar, or glycerine over a period of time and then straining, in order to extract the medicinal compounds.

Vermifuge An agent that rids the body of worms (anthelmintic).

Vulnerary A remedy that promotes healing of wounds.

BIBLIOGRAPHY

Boxer, Arabella and Philippa Back. *The Herb Book.* London: Octopus Books Limited, 1981.

Buhner, Stephen Harrod. *Sacred Plant Medicine: The Wisdom in Native American Herbalism.* Rochester, VT: Bear & Company, 2006.

Bunney, Sarah. *The Illustrated Encyclopedia of Herbs, Their Medicinal and Culinary Uses.* London: Chancellor Press, 1992.

Burke, Nancy. *The Modern Herbal Primer, A Simple Guide to the Magic and Medicine of 100 Healing Herbs.* Alexandria, Virginia: Time-Life Books (Old Farmer's Almanac Home Library), 2000.

Castleman, Michael. *The Healing Herbs, The Ultimate Guide to the Curative Power of Nature's Medicines.* Emmaus, Pennsylvania: Rodale Press, 1991.

Clough, Katherine. *Wildflowers of Prince Edward Island.* Charlottetown, PEI: Ragweed Press, 1995.

Duke, James A. *The Green Pharmacy.* Emmaus, Pennsylvania: Rodale Press, 1997.

Easley, Thomas and Steven Horne. *The Modern Herbal Dispensary, A Medicine-Making Guide.* Berkeley, California: North Atlantic Books, 2016

Foster, Steven and Rebecca L. Johnson. *Desk Reference to Nature's Medicine.* Washington, DC: National Geographic Society, 2006.

Foster, Steven and James A. Duke. *Eastern/Central Medicinal Plants and Herbs of Eastern and Central North America.* New York: Houghton Mifflin Company (Peterson Field Guide Series), 2000.

Gray, Beverley. *The Boreal Herbal, Wild Food and Medicine of the North.* Whitehorse, Yukon: Aroma Borealis Press, Co-published by Canadian Circumpolar Institute, 2011.

Grieve, Maud. *A Modern Herbal.* London: Tiger Books International, 1973 (originally published in 1931).

Hoffmann, David. *The Complete Illustrated Holistic Herbal.* London: Element (An Imprint of Harper Collins), 2002.

Kloos, Scott. *Pacific Northwest Medicinal Plants.* Portland, Oregon: Timber Press, Inc., 2017.

Lacey, Laurie. *Mi'kmaq Medicines, Remedies and Recollections.* Halifax, NS: Nimbus Publishing, 2012.

MacKinnon, Andrew A. *Edible & Medicinal Plants of Canada.* Edmonton, Alberta: Partners Publishing, and Lone Pine Media Productions (BC), 2014.

Pahlow, Mannfried. *Healing Plants.* Hauppauge, NY: Barron's Educational Series, Inc., 1993.

Redfield, Edmund. *Wildflowers of the Maritimes: A Guide to Identifying 150 of the Region's Wild Plants.* Halifax, NS: Nimbus Publishing, 2016.

Reader's Digest. *Magic and Medicine of Plants.* Pleasantville, New York: Reader's Digest Association, Inc., 1989.

Scott, Peter J. *Edible Plants of Atlantic Canada.* Portugal Cove-St. Philip's, Newfoundland and Labrador: Boulder Publications, 2010.

Tierra, Michael. *The Way of Herbs.* New York: Pocket Books (Simon and Shuster), 1998.

Vermeulen, Nico. *The Complete Encyclopedia of Herbs.* Lisse, The Netherlands: Rebo Publishers, 1998.

Walker, Marilyn. *Wild Plants of Eastern Canada.* Halifax, NS: Nimbus Publishing, 2008.

Wood, Matthew. *The Earthwise Herbal Repertory.* Berkeley, California: North Atlantic Books, 2016.